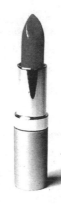

DROP-DEAD GORGEOUS

Protecting Yourself from the Hidden Dangers of Cosmetics

KIM ERICKSON	Foreword by Samuel S. Epstein, M.D., author of *The Safe Shopper's Bible*

Contemporary Books

Chicago   New York   San Francisco   Lisbon   London   Madrid   Mexico City
Milan   New Delhi   San Juan   Seoul   Singapore   Sydney   Toronto

Library of Congress Cataloging-in-Publication Data

Erickson, Kim.
    Drop-dead gorgeous : protecting yourself from the hidden dangers of
cosmetics / Kim Erickson ; foreword by Samuel S. Epstein, M.D.
        p.   cm.
    Includes index.
    ISBN 0-658-01793-4 (alk. paper)
      1. Cosmetics—Toxicology.   2. Toilet preparations—Toxicology.
3. Women—Health and hygiene.   4. Consumer education.   I. Title.

RA1270.C65 E75   2002
363.19′6—dc21   2001047838

Contemporary Books

A Division of The **McGraw·Hill** *Companies*

1 2 3 4 5 6 7 8 9 0   AGM/AGM   1 0 9 8 7 6 5 4 3 2

ISBN 0-658-01793-4

This book was set in Minion.
Printed and bound by Quebecor Martinsburg

Cover design by Nick Panos
Cover photograph copyright © Jill Birschbach
Interior design by Susan H. Hartman

McGraw-Hill books are available at special quantity discounts to use as premiums and sales promotions, or for use in corporate training programs. For more information, please write to the Director of Special Sales, Professional Publishing, McGraw-Hill, Two Penn Plaza, New York, NY 10121-2298. Or contact your local bookstore.

This book is printed on acid-free paper.

For my grandmother,
whose independent spirit and love of beauty
were a true inspiration.

Like the constant dripping of water that in turn wears away the hardest stone, this birth-to-death contact with dangerous chemicals may in the end prove disastrous. Each of these recurrent exposures, no matter how slight, contributes to the progressive build up of chemicals in our bodies and so to cumulative poisoning.

Lulled by the soft sell and the hidden persuader, the average citizen is seldom aware of the deadly materials with which he is surrounding himself; indeed, he may not realize he is using them at all.

—Rachel Carson, *Silent Spring*

Contents

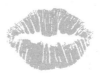

Foreword

Drop-Dead Gorgeous couldn't be more aptly named. Mainstream industry cosmetics and personal care products are witches' brews of carcinogens without any warning on their labels. The great majority of adult women, in addition to men, can use a dozen or so products a day; some products are also widely used on infants and children. Thus, exposure to these products is virtually lifelong, from birth to death. Some products are applied to large areas of skin on which they can remain for extended periods. Many product ingredients are readily absorbed through the skin, and absorption is increased by harsh detergent ingredients, particularly sodium lauryl sulfate. As such, mainstream industry products represent the single largest class of involuntary and avoidable carcinogenic exposures. This is critical in view of the escalating incidence of cancer, which has now reached epidemic proportions, striking one in every two men and one in every three women in their lifetimes, and with some 550,000 estimated cancer deaths in 2001. This is even more critical in view of the fact that consumers have an inalienable right to know of information vital to their health and safety, although such information remains buried in government and industry files or in the relatively inaccessible scientific literature.

In her reader-friendly and meticulously documented book, Kim Erickson guides consumers on how to read and interpret the poorly informative listings of ingredients on product labels. She then presents comprehensive information on mainstream industry ingredients, based largely on information about the products of named individual companies detailed in the 1995 *Safe Shopper's Bible*, which I coauthored. Erickson identifies ingredients that are carcinogenic themselves, as well as those that are contaminated by carcinogens, that are precursors of carcinogens, or that break down to form carcinogens. Examples include "frank" carcinogens such as talc and the surfactant DEA; other surfactants such as PEG, contaminated with the volatile carcinogen 1,4-dioxane, which could easily be removed during the manufacturing process by simple vacuum stripping; nitrite, or nitrite derived from bronopol, reacting with DEA as a precursor of the carcinogenic nitrosamine (NDELA), as has been well-known since the mid-1970s; and imidazolidinyl urea, which is broken down in the bottle itself or in the skin to release the carcinogenic formaldehyde. Erickson particularly warns against risks of ovarian cancer from genital dusting with talc by young women and risks of relatively rare cancers, non-Hodgkin's lymphoma, multiple myeloma, and leukemia, along with ovarian cancer from the regular use of black or dark brown permanent or semipermanent hair dyes. Erickson also identifies a wide range of ingredients posing other toxic hazards, including irritant, allergic, neurotoxic, reproductive, and endocrine disruptive effects.

This book, however, is not a "sky-is-falling-in" tale of woe, as Erickson offers extensive recipes for do-it-yourself safe alternatives. These include shopping and formulating instructions suitable for any kitchen. While preparation of some recipes may be relatively labor intensive, this commitment is more than counterbalanced by the products' low costs as well as their safety, for which the overwhelming majority of consumers would be prepared to pay a premium.

For the majority of consumers who would rather purchase retail products, the book provides useful information on sources of alternative safe products in the text and appendixes. This is not an easy matter. As Erickson strongly cautions, a wide range of alternative or nonmainstream companies tout themselves as "green" or "organic," in some instances by simply adding a few organic ingredients to a soup of synthetic and often other hazardous ingredients. The largest and most deceptive of these "greenwashers" is Anita Roddick's The Body Shop, which proclaims its dedication to organic principles and safety, as well as to progressive and altruistic ideology, although its product ingredients are barely, if at all, distinguishable from those used by mainstream industries. In contrast to such greenwashers, Erickson recommends Aubrey Organics, whose products are available on a relatively limited basis in health food stores. Aubrey claims that it uses a majority of organic ingredients in all of its products; however, of eight products recently reviewed, only three contained one of two defined or certified organic ingredients—aloe and jojoba oil. More widely available recommended safe products are those of Aveda and Neways International. Aveda, with approximately two thousand national and international salons and other outlets, was recently acquired by Estée Lauder. Aveda's fragrances have, since the company's inception in 1978, been entirely organic. Over the last few years, Aveda has also made remarkable progress in phasing out carcinogenic and other synthetic ingredients from its products. Neways International, a multilevel marketing industry, operating worldwide through a network of distributors, is also phasing out its carcinogenic ingredients, under guidance of the Cancer Prevention Coalition. These companies are experiencing rapid growth and may well pose a future challenge, or even serve as an example, to mainstream industries.

Erickson believes that beauty is not skin deep, that it reflects self-esteem, spirituality, and holistic principles, to all of which she devotes a significant segment of the book. While to some this may be of questionable relevance, I find it complementary to her concerns about safety and an unexpected bonus in the book.

Such a prodigious book as *Drop-Dead Gorgeous* cannot possibly be totally criticism-free. One concern relates to its extensive focus on women. While in most traditional families, women do the shopping, including for cosmetics and personal care products or for do-it-yourself ingredients, an increasing proportion of U.S. families is now composed of single women and, to a lesser extent, of single males, apart from the increasing proportion of unmarried, late marrying, or homosexual males. So, surely more emphasis should have been directed to cosmetics and personal care products used by men, who receive only trivial reference in the book. Also, emphasis should have been directed to the use of personal care products for infants and children, who are more susceptible than adults to carcinogens and other toxicants.

One final concern relates to the Food and Drug Administration. Erickson takes the position that the major reason why the FDA is so ineffective in regulating cosmetics is its inadequate budget. While this concern cannot be dismissed, in fact, the major reason is the FDA's track record of unwillingness or disinterest in implementing the 1938 Federal Food, Drug, and Cosmetic Act, along with the Fair Packaging Labeling Act. These acts give the agency full authority to declare as "misbranded" any product containing ingredients harmful to consumers. Once "misbranded," the product is subject to regulatory action, including seizure and recall, authority that the FDA has rarely invoked. Instead, the agency periodically expresses "serious concern" regarding carcinogenic ingredients, evidence on some of which has been well documented for decades. Thus, the major problem of the continued marketing of hazardous products by the mainstream industry is the FDA's reckless regulatory abdication, compounded by industry's unresponsiveness.

Minor criticisms aside, Erickson must be congratulated on having written a superb and up-to-date book that should grace the homes of all Americans, apart from consumers in other major industrialized nations. This book should be a bestseller.

—Samuel S. Epstein, M.D.
Professor emeritus, environmental and occupational medicine,
University of Illinois School of Public Health, Chicago,
and chairman, Cancer Prevention Coalition

Acknowledgments

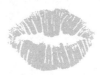

Nothing is created in a void. Over the course of writing this book I have received help and encouragement from numerous people who generously shared their time, talents, and expertise. I would especially like to thank those people who reviewed portions of the manuscript: Susan Haeger, the former executive director of Citizens for Health, as well as Dr. Joseph Coffineau and Michelle De Fazio of the National Toxic Encephalopathy Foundation. Dave DeRosa of the Greenpeace Toxics Campaign deserves special mention for looking through a confused first draft and offering numerous suggestions.

In addition, my special appreciation to the following for their advice and interviews: Dr. Steve Allen Jr. of the State University of New York, Pat Costner of Greenpeace, Dr. Joel Goodman of The Humor Project, Inc., Dr. Elson Haas of the Preventive Medical Center of Marin, Dr. Theo Kruck of the University of Toronto (ret.), Dr. Steven Lamm of the New York University School of Medicine, Dr. Lorraine Meisner, Dr. William Pendlebury of the University of Vermont, Dr. Gary Spencer, and Dr. David Stoll. I would also like to thank the women whose stories appear in these pages and all of the others who asked that their stories be kept private.

I am also indebted to the following experts, whose writings provided background for this book: James and Phyllis Balch, Rachael Carson, Dr. Theo Colborn, James Duke, Dianne Dumanoski, Stephen Edelson, Dr. Samuel Epstein, Dan Fagin, Lois Marie Gibbs, Aubrey Hampton, Annette Huddle,

Kathi Keville, Marianne Lavelle, Dr. John Peterson Myers, Sheldon Rampton, Dr. Ted Schettler, Dr. Gina Solomon, David Steinman, John Stauber, Maria Valenti, Judi Vance, and Ruth Winter. Of course, none of this would be possible without the scientists and consumer advocates upon whose tireless, and often underfunded, work this book is based.

Thanks also go to Peter Hoffman for believing in the book and Claudia McCowan for her early editorial guidance. A very special thank-you goes to my editor at Contemporary Books, Betsy Lane, who was always there with enthusiastic advice and skillful editorial guidance. Lynn Prowitt-Smith and Vera Tweed of GreatLife magazine also deserve my gratitude for publishing articles based on information that eventually went into creating this book, as does Jim Motavalli of *E: The Environmental Magazine.*

Finally, to my friends and family, whose encouragement has sustained me throughout this long journey—particularly my parents, whose unwavering love and support were more than any daughter could ask for; my sister, Julie, for her constant enthusiasm; and Jane and Frank, whose faith gave me the courage to keep working—you'll never know how grateful I am. To Brandon and Whitney, who always supported me despite the ups and downs of having a freelance writer for a mother. And to my husband, Mike. Your constant encouragement and unconditional love are the cornerstones of my life.

Introduction

Every morning, millions of American women naively reach for the shampoo, conditioner, moisturizer, and deodorant. Without giving it a second thought, we diligently spritz, spray, paint, and powder, blissfully unaware that this daily ritual exposes us to more than two hundred synthetic chemicals—and all before our morning coffee!

For years, the hazards of cosmetics and personal care products were the best-kept secret in consumer goods. Even today, cosmetics safety doesn't get a lot of play in the media. With few exceptions, it is an issue usually classified as "fluff." New research warning us of the dangers that modern cosmetics pose is virtually ignored. Consequently, most women have no idea that cosmetics have a less-than-benign alter ego—one that can have potentially deadly consequences.

Environmental health and consumer advocacy groups aren't paying much attention either. Compared with the toxins found in our air, soil, and waterways, cosmetics seem a trivial pursuit. Yet, many of the same poisons that pollute our environment—from dioxin to petrochemicals—can be found in the jars and bottles that line our bathroom shelves.

While it's too early to know with any certainty how serious the long-term health impacts will be, the warning signs are ominous. Many of the ingredients found in modern cosmetics have been identified as hazardous by the U.S. Environmental Protection Agency. Scientists caution that hormone-disrupting chemicals may lurk in cosmetics; these chemicals could lower our immunity to disease and cause neurological and reproductive damage. Many of these same ingredients have been found to cause cancer in laboratory animals and, in some cases, humans. At best, a visit to your neighborhood cosmetics counter could result in allergies, irritations, and sensitivities.

Why are our makeup bags filled with this hazardous waste? Because synthetic chemicals are inexpensive, are stable, and have a long shelf life. The bottom line is that cosmetics manufacturers, and their stockholders, enjoy the profitability provided by the ever-growing variety of synthetic ingredients.

Whatever happened to natural cosmetics—nontoxic products that are actually good for you? Makeup mavens say they don't exist. According to consumer advocate Paula Begoun, author of *The Beauty Bible*, "There is no such thing as all-natural, pure cosmetics." Although these products may not be available at the cosmetics counters and drugstores where she shops, they can be had. That's what this book is all about.

One note about the shopping guides found in the following chapters: While every effort has been made to find effective nontoxic cosmetics, some of the products listed do contain synthetic ingredients. Check the list of ingredients on the label before you buy *any* cosmetics or personal care products.

Part I	What's Really in Your Cosmetics?

1
Our Synthetic Society

"Most cosmetic manufacturers will use any kind of slogan to make you disregard their ingredients."
—Aubrey Hampton

Almost from the moment of our arrival on the planet, we humans have been preoccupied with trying to improve the package we came in. Our fascination with color and appreciation of beauty are part of our nature, carrying with them an almost instinctive desire to enhance our own appearance. We know that looking good not only makes us more attractive to others but also makes us feel good about ourselves.

So, we primp, we perm, we powder—all without blinking a mascara-swathed eye. After all, we have laws and government agencies to assure that the products we use on our hair and skin are safe, right? Don't be too sure. Modern cosmetics contain a host of dubious ingredients that sound as if they'd be more at home in a test tube than on our faces. And although, for most of us, the majority of products appear safe in the short run, the results from long-term use could be deadly. Coal tar colors, phenylenediamine, benzene, even formaldehyde, are just a few of the synthetic chemicals commonly included in shampoos, skin creams, and blushes—toxins that are absorbed into your skin with every use.

During the past fifty years, science and big business have teamed up to bring a steady stream of new and "better" products to consumers, many of them aimed at our desire for instant beauty. With systems working at breakneck speed, and with billions of dollars at stake, the primary aim of this alliance was to protect the cosmetics trade. This method of ensuring continued industry profits and consumer demand was a strategy that worked well for many years. But during the 1970s, consumers began to question the safety of mainstream cosmetics. To counteract the growing skepticism on the part of consumers, manufacturers set out to prove how safe their products were by sponsoring research into several of the synthetic chemicals commonly found in cosmetics. While the results sounded reassuring, the politics and science behind the studies were anything but. Since the studies were paid for by the cosmetics companies, it was no surprise that the findings ultimately supported the industry's profit margin by using misleading research to soothe consumer's fears.

The few independent studies that have been conducted have resulted in some alarming findings. A recent report from Xavier University in Louisiana found high levels of lead in Grecian Formula and Lady Grecian Formula hair dyes—so much that researchers weren't able to wash it off their hands after using the product![1] Another study reported that women who color their hair show greater chromosomal damage than women who have never used hair dyes.[2] And Swedish researchers have found that allergic reactions to nail polish included lesions that covered the face, neck, and hands of test subjects sensitive to toluene-sulfonamide/formaldehyde resin.[3]

Although sporadic independent research continues, consumers are rarely privy to the findings. These studies, conducted without the benefit of industry backing, usually appear buried in obscure medical journals and gain little attention from the media. Those that do make the headlines are disputed by industry-funded experts who make the findings appear false or inconclusive. This scientific "he said, she said" scenario makes it all but impossible for consumers to understand the impact that modern cosmetics can have on their health.

The Lure of Advertising

Despite mounting evidence that cosmetics can be hazardous to our health, new products continue to find their way into our bathrooms and boudoirs. In a culture based on youth and beauty, we're buying more cosmetics than ever before in an attempt to erase the years, enhance what's lacking, and fit in with the elusive and ever-changing Madison Avenue standard of the perfect woman. As Rita Freedman notes in her book *Beauty Bound,* "The daily beauty fix can be as addictive, compelling, and expensive as some drug habits."[4] It's certainly profitable for the cosmetics industry, whose sales have grown from $7 billion in 1970 to a whopping $28 billion in 1994.[5]

With so much money at stake, the cosmetics industry makes it its business to pinpoint and exploit the hopes, fears, and insecurities American women have when it comes to our looks. They know we are aging. They know we face a crossroads between careerism and traditional femininity. They know we have more disposable income, and they want us to spend it on their products. To assure growing industry sales, advertisers target the anxiety that swirls around our physical appearance, spinning a fairy tale of beauty and sex appeal that begins the moment we reach puberty. Stacked up against advertisers' computer-enhanced fashion models, our own flaws—real and imagined—jump out at us. These fears and insecurities blossom into what we come to perceive as need. It's a need cosmetics manufacturers are all too happy to fill via a constant bombardment of advertising campaigns that promise radiant hair and flawless skin. In fact, cosmetics companies are the largest of all television and print advertisers, targeting not only the traditional eighteen- to thirty-five-year-old market but also the 75 million baby boomers[6] trying to defy the effects of time.

In today's competitive marketplace, developing a successful sales pitch isn't left to mere chance. Since the end of World War II, marketing unnecessary necessities has become a science of statistics. Marketing gurus comb the latest research. Demographics are studied—including age, gender, race, marital status, where you live, even where you shop and what you buy. Census data, market patterns, and behavioral research are all compiled and dissected. But instead of improving their products to reflect consumers' true wants and needs, the industry simply uses this data to refine the sales pitch. The resulting ad campaign isn't designed to appeal to the reality of consumers' lives but to the fears and fantasies the industry has created. In the world of beauty, that means a subtle, yet in-your-face, barrage of messages delivered by gorgeous, anorexic eighteen-year-olds who flicker across our TV screens or are captured between the covers of the latest fashion magazine. The message is clear: if you use this product, you can look like me. The hype is so successful that we've become a culture preoccupied with an illusion—and we'll pay any price to attain it. We *want* to believe.

We've all succumbed to the illusion at one time or another. If you think you're immune, take this simple test: Look in your makeup drawer. If you're like most women, you may be astonished to find dozens of lipsticks, eye shadows, blushers, creams, and lotions—each one promising instant beauty, and many of which are barely used. In this era of overconsumption, most American households contain at least two kinds of soap, three kinds of toothpaste, and a half dozen different colognes. Do we really *need* all those synthetic products to keep us fresh and alluring, or are we just being manipulated for someone else's gain?

The Greenwashing Game

In today's health-conscious market, touting a product's naturalness can turn a "ho-hum" product into a top seller. Running a close second are the feel-good claims of environmentalism and social responsibility. Products ranging from ice cream to long-distance telephone services have successfully turned these worthy values into higher profits—and the cosmetics industry is clamoring to get in on the action. Using aggressive, well-funded public relations and marketing campaigns, these companies can give themselves the *appearance* of caring about consumers' health and the health of the planet while still protecting conventional manufacturing practices—and consequently their bottom line.

Positioning a company as "green" isn't anything new. Just ask Anita Roddick, owner of The Body Shop, who has parlayed environmentalism and social conscience into more than eighteen hundred stores worldwide.[7] Roddick discovered early on that public relations could help her products stand out from the crowd by linking herself with third-world economics, progressive social programs, and the growing interest in natural products. To that end, The Body Shop has promoted itself by using raw materials from such diverse locations as Bangladesh, Nepal, Zambia, and the Amazon through its "Trade Not Aid" (now called "Community Trade") program—a program supposedly designed to help indigenous people build better lives for themselves through the sale of exotic cosmetics ingredients.[8] "In a cassette version of her autobiography, titled *Body and Soul: Profits with Principles*, . . . Roddick claims: 'We simply and honestly sell wholesome products that women want. We sell them at reasonable prices without exploiting anyone, without hurting animals, without hurting the earth. We do it all without lying, cheating, and without even advertising.'"[9] Yet, during an investigative report for National Public Radio, journalist Jon Entine found that only a small fraction of the ingredients The Body Shop used came from Trade Not

Aid and many of its products relied on outdated formulas filled with non-renewable, less-than-natural petrochemicals.[10] In fact, a quick survey of the company's 2001 cosmetics line reveals an overwhelming number of synthetic—potentially dangerous—ingredients, including sodium laureth sulfate, cocamide DEA, polyvinylpyrrolidone (PVP), and benzalkonium chloride, not to mention synthetic colors and an alphabet soup of preservatives. Worse yet, the company has a history of selling products contaminated with formaldehyde.[11]

In spite of these facts, the company continues to spin a fairy tale for consumers and investors alike. In the face of disappointing profits in 2001, the company's CEO, Patrick Gournay, assured investors that The Body Shop has become an authority on developing unique personal care products based on natural ingredients drawn from a diversity of cultural knowledge from around the world and plans to continue its market growth with honesty and integrity.[12]

But one group that hasn't bought into The Body Shop's self-proclaimed image is the London chapter of Greenpeace. The group has organized demonstrations in protest of the company's business practices, claiming: "Behind the green and cuddly image lies the reality—The Body Shop's operations, like those of all multinationals, have a detrimental effect on the environment and the world's poor. They do not help the plight of animals or indigenous peoples and their products are far from what they're cracked up to be." The group goes on to charge The Body Shop with placing itself on a pedestal in order to exploit people's idealism.[13] Even as Roddick asks consumers to investigate "the story behind the label," her own empire's "green" image is withering under the microscope.

Yet, not all multinational cosmetics companies subscribe to business as usual. One company that appears to be bucking the status quo is Aveda. Founded in 1978 by Horst Rechelbacher, Aveda offers one thousand–plus products through its more than fifteen hundred salons and select outlets worldwide.[14] Although Aveda has positioned itself as a socially responsible company with strong environmental principles, the company had historically used synthetic ingredients as a base for the botanicals it often touted in its marketing literature. But, after becoming a subsidiary of cosmetics giant Estée Lauder in 1998—a strange union indeed—some unexpected changes began to occur. In a bold move, Aveda launched a global reformulation program in 1999 and began phasing out many of the synthetic ingredients on which it had relied for so long. Among the first ingredients targeted were diazolidinyl urea and talc. Aveda has also enlisted independent evaluations from outside the company to identify other suspect ingredients.

Although it will take some time to complete the transition to safer ingredients, Aveda seems committed. The company has launched a line of synthetic-free fragrances and is concentrating on nonanimal safety testing at its in-house Safety Lab.[15] And, unlike The Body Shop, which lines its shelves with plastic containers, Aveda packages its products in 10 to 30 percent recycled glass whenever practical.[16] In fact, Aveda uses more recycled material for its packaging than any other company in America.[17]

While it would be premature to classify Aveda as a truly natural cosmetics company, it is encouraging to see this major industry player take action without the self-instigated fanfare so common in the industry. If Aveda succeeds, it will be the consumer who profits.

The Cosmetics Industry's Other Face

The cosmetics industry would like us to believe that it has our best interests at heart, particularly when it comes to the safety of its products. But the truth isn't so reassuring. Thanks to weak, ineffective consumer regulation, the cosmetics industry is in the enviable position of policing itself— and it's the job of the Cosmetic, Toiletry, and Fragrance Association (CTFA) to keep it that way. The CTFA is the industry's trade organization, a powerful special-interest group designed to protect the industry, not the consumer. The vast majority of cosmetics companies in the United States rely on the CTFA's lobbyists to refute scientific studies that show that the ingredients used in hair dyes, lipsticks, and skin creams are potentially dangerous.

Although CTFA president E. Edward Kavanaugh insists that cosmetics are absolutely safe and that additional safety testing isn't necessary,[18] public health advocates disagree and would like to see the Food and Drug Administration (FDA) awarded more money for research and more authority to regulate the industry. Vigorously opposing such action, the CTFA uses its powerful political action committee to maintain the status quo with members of Congress.

One member of Congress who isn't sold is former representative Ron Wyden, a Democrat from Oregon, who introduced a bill that would have required cosmetics manufacturers to list the ingredients on the products used by professional cosmetologists, especially hair dyes. When the legislation failed, one congressional staff member reportedly said: "Until further action is taken, women are worse off than guinea pigs. At least with guinea pigs, someone is watching."[19]

Ethics and the Environment

The risks of synthetic chemicals extend beyond human health. Many of the ingredients in cosmetics are environmental pollutants. Along with the waste produced during the manufacturing process, millions of gallons of synthetic chemicals are washed down the drain and into sewer systems every day. Petrochemicals commonly used in makeup, skin creams, and hair care products not only contaminate our waterways but also can destroy marine life. Several studies have shown high levels of benzene and naphthalene in the brain tissue of rainbow trout and coho salmon.[20] The surfactants in hair rinses, shampoos, and lotions can end up in the soil, significantly changing the way plants grow.[21] And the production of acetic acid and ethylene glycol, ingredients found in many lotions and hair dyes, contributes to air pollution.

It's not just the raw materials that cause concern but also the by-products produced as these chemicals degrade. The breakdown of some of the ingredients found in personal care products can result in alkylphenol ethoxylate surfactants. These surfactants interfere with the normal functioning of hormones and may confuse sexual development. Alkylphenol ethoxylates generally end up in sewage treatment plants, where they degrade into other alkylphenolic compounds. Eventually making their way into our rivers and seas, these substances create a persistent threat to wildlife. Even small amounts of alkylphenolic compounds are dangerous since these substances become concentrated in the internal organs of fish and birds at levels up to ten times greater than those found in the surrounding environment.[22]

For years, scientists and environmentalists have warned of the devastating effects these hormone disruptors can have in nature. They cite the salmon in Lake Erie that were discovered to have greatly enlarged thyroid glands— up to a million times the normal size. And at the Saint Lawrence Estuary in Quebec, a beluga whale was found to have two testicles and two separate sets of ovaries. Between 1985 and 1990, 67 percent of the male panthers in the

Florida Everglades were found to have undescended testes, low sperm counts, and abnormal sperm.[23]

Scientists also speculate that dioxin, a by-product of some manufacturing processes, impairs the immune system of certain mammals. They point to the massive die-off of seals in the North and Baltic Seas and of dolphins along the eastern seaboard. Studies of seals fed dioxin-contaminated fish showed a significantly lower immune response than seals fed a less contaminated diet.[24] Exposure to dioxin can also cause cancers, birth defects, and fetal death in domestic and wild animals.

Even though numerous independent studies have documented the health and environmental consequences of dioxins, many industrial chemists disagree. Their argument is that because dioxins are ubiquitous, we need not be concerned about them. Yet, tossed into landfills, these dioxins leach into the soil and water, eventually settling into the fatty tissues of fish and animals.

Unfortunately, environmental damage doesn't stop with what's *in* the bottle or jar you pick up off the store shelf. Attractive packaging may be an integral part of the cosmetics industry's marketing strategy, but disposing of this excessive packaging contributes to the problem of our ever-shrinking landfills. In fact, product packaging accounts for nearly 30 percent of the trash disposed of each year.[25]

In addition to creating more solid waste, compounds found in plastic shampoo bottles and in skin cream jars, as well as chlorine-bleached cardboard boxes and the paper used for package inserts, can leach toxic substances into soil and groundwater. As these toxins eventually work their way back into our food and water supply, we become victims of our own consumption.

But perhaps the most immediate victims of synthetic cosmetics are the animals routinely used for safety testing. Mahatma Gandhi once observed that "the greatness of a nation and its moral progress can be judged by the way its animals are treated." Yet, between 10 million and 15 million animals are tortured and killed every year in American laboratories in an attempt to determine the safety of cosmetics and household products.[26] In addition to the rats, mice, and guinea pigs we normally think of in laboratory settings, dogs, cats, rabbits, and even primates are subjected to inhumane testing procedures, often without the benefit of anesthetics or analgesics—pain relievers that might interfere with the test results.

An assortment of tests designed to measure skin irritancy and damage due to inhalation are routinely conducted on experimental animals, but the most insidious are the Draize Eye Irritancy Test and the LD50 test.

The Draize test, invented in 1944, is used to test products such as mascara and shampoos for eye irritation and tissue damage. Rabbits are restrained in stocks, and metal clips hold their eyes open while drops, flakes, or granules of the concentrated chemical or product being tested are placed in the lower lid of each eye. Damage is measured by the amount of swelling, redness, and irritation that occurs over a seven-day period. During the test, these animals can suffer extreme burning, swelling, hemorrhaging, lacerations of the iris, and ultimately blindness.[27]

LD50 stands for Lethal Dose 50 Percent. This test measures how much of a compound is needed to kill 50 percent of the group of laboratory animals selected for the test—often dogs, cats, pigs, or monkeys. Ingredients routinely used in nail polish, hair dye, lipstick, perfume, and skin creams are force-fed to the test animals over a period ranging from two weeks to seven years, depending on the compound. Once the tolerance level of a chemical has been reached, the animals can experience loss of appetite, diarrhea, vomiting, convulsions, and bleeding from the eyes, nose, and mouth before finally dying.[28]

With the exception of previously untested color additives, current laws administered by the FDA do not require the use of animal testing for cosmetics,[29] nor are they considered reliable indicators of product safety. According to Dr. Herbert Gundersheimer of the Physicians Committee for Responsible Medicine, "Results of animal tests are not transferable between species, and therefore cannot guarantee product safety for humans."[30] The cosmetics industry's trade publication, *Drug and Cosmetic Industry*, even admits that "no animal has skin which closely resembles human skin, neither anatomically nor physiologically."[31]

Although it is generally accepted that nonanimal testing is faster and more economical, movement toward a more humane form of testing by cosmetics manufacturers is slow. One company resisting the trend toward more humane testing is Procter & Gamble, the manufacturer of Cover Girl, Max Factor, and Vidal Sassoon brands. Even though Procter & Gamble spends millions of dollars distributing promotional materials heralding its efforts to eliminate animal testing, it's all smoke and mirrors. In 1993 alone, Procter & Gamble invested $2.4 *billion* on advertising while spending only $450,000 in scientific grants to develop actual alternatives to animal testing.[32] When asked if it planned to stop animal testing, Procter & Gamble responded that it had no plans to alter current policy in the foreseeable future. Until Procter & Gamble abandons this double standard, In Defense of Animals, an animal rights group based in Mill Valley, California, is spearheading a nationwide boycott of all P&G products.[33]

Procter & Gamble isn't alone in continuing this barbaric practice. Other industry giants such as Alberto-Culver, Coty, and Unilever[34] still persist in conducting animal testing. If live animal testing is neither required nor reliable, why do these companies continue to count on it for product safety? According to the Physicians Committee for Responsible Medicine, "It appears that testing is part of the process by which manufacturers avoid legal liability for damages caused by their products."[35] Fortunately, animal rights groups are successfully shining the light on the dark secret of animal testing. The pressure is on as a greater segment of the public consciously seeks out products that have not been tested on animals.

Reinventing the Ritual

While we may not be able to depend on the government or the cosmetics industry to protect us from the toxins commonly found in cosmetics, we can learn to protect ourselves. The last decade has proved to be one of growing individual involvement in our own health and well-being. We exercise, we meditate, and alternative medicine has gone mainstream. The intense consumerism and "do-it-all" superwoman mentality that defined the 1980s have given way to a more balanced awareness of health and wholeness for ourselves and the environment in which we live. We're taking better care of ourselves by taking charge of our own lives.

As we become more health conscious, it's important that we learn the truth about the consequences of our choices—not just concerning the foods we eat or how stress affects our well-being, but also how our daily beauty routines impact our health. Although discovering what's really in the products in which we lavishly indulge day in and day out can be frightening and frustrating, it's an education with a happy ending—one you can instigate yourself. In the face of high-priced, chemically packed, and potentially harmful cosmetics, we can reinvent the healthful, soul-satisfying ritual of beauty that our ancestors knew so well.

Toxic Beauty

"Beautiful to look on, contaminating to the touch."
—*The Malleus Maleficarum*, 1486

Looking at Denise Santamarina, you'd never suspect that this petite, perky blond has spent the past ten years battling chemically induced lupus. "I started getting sick when I began taking cosmetology classes," says the thirty-four-year-old cosmetologist. "Over the next ten years, I suffered from a string of digestive problems, sinus infections, and excruciating pain in my back, rib cage, and arms. There were days when I would crawl across the floor, almost as if I were trying to crawl out of my body and away from the pain." Most of the doctors who saw Denise merely treated her symptoms or dismissed her complaints as stress related. Neither she nor the doctors made any connection between her medical problems and the scores of chemicals to which she was exposed in her job until a chemical screening showed high levels of benzene and toluene—both common ingredients in nail polish and polish remover.

Instead of giving in to the disease, Denise decided to fight back. Taking responsibility for her own health, she quit her job as a manicurist, tossed out all the chemically laced cosmetics stashed under her bathroom sink, and adopted a healthy lifestyle. She began working with a nutritionist to detoxify her system and switched to an organically based diet. Over the next few years, Denise educated herself in natural alternatives to synthetic hair, skin, and nail care. Today, she's a whirlwind of activity, juggling a husband and three children. Still drawn to a career in beauty, Denise now operates a nontoxic salon and spa in Las Vegas to meet the needs of clients suffering from chemical sensitivities or those simply concerned with a more healthful beauty experience. "Looking good shouldn't compromise your health," says Denise, who offers her patrons a full range of services using only natural ingredients.

What happened to Denise is rare. The sudden onset of violent symptoms isn't a typical profile of chemical poisoning. For most of us, the adverse health effects of toxins compound over the course of several decades, confusing our hormone receptors and slowly altering our cell structure. The resulting cancer may not appear for twenty or thirty years.

Today, we are exposed to synthetic chemicals in every facet of our lives. Rachel Carson alerted us to this trend toward a synthetic world nearly fifty years ago in her classic book, *Silent Spring*: "For the first time in the history of the world, every human being is now subjected to contact with dangerous chemicals from the moment of conception to death."[1] But could Carson have imagined the speed at which synthetic chemicals are being introduced today? The United Nations Environmental Programme estimates that approximately seventy thousand chemicals are currently in common use, with a thousand new chemicals being introduced every year.[2] Many of these find their way onto store shelves in cosmetics and personal care products. Of all the chemicals used in cosmetics, the National Institute of Occupational Safety and Health has reported that nearly nine hundred are toxic.[3]

Protection Under the Law?

When the Federal Food, Drug, and Cosmetic Act was passed by Congress in 1938, it was intended to ensure the purity and safety of food, drugs, and cosmetics products. Unfortunately for consumers, this all-inclusive blanket of protection has some very large holes in it, especially when it comes to cosmetics.

While most of us assume that the Food and Drug Administration employs hundreds of scientists in little white coats to protect us from the harmful ingredients in our cosmetics, the truth is far less reassuring. Falling under the jurisdiction of the U.S. Congress, the FDA is charged with monitoring the safety of every morsel we eat and every drug on the market, both over-the-counter and prescription, not to mention the scores of medical devices available. Pitted against these critical consumer goods, cosmetics fall somewhere around the bottom of the agency's pecking order and consequently receive the lowest priority when it comes to regulatory power and funding.

As the FDA's stepchild under the current system, cosmetics can be regulated only after they appear in the marketplace. Unlike food or drugs, cosmetics products and the raw ingredients they contain aren't subject to review or premarket approval before being sold to the public. What's more, manufacturers aren't required to report cosmetics-related injuries or submit safety data on the ingredients used in their products.[4]

Already underfunded and understaffed, the FDA's Office of Cosmetics and Colors (OCC) was hit with budget cuts in 1998, resulting in employee layoffs and the untimely death of several critical programs. In the face of these cuts, the OCC suspended testing for the presence of carcinogens in products and shut down a program that encouraged manufacturers of cosmetics to voluntarily provide data on their products—a program in which more than half of all manufacturers participated.

Fortunately, Congress reversed itself with the FDA's 1999 fiscal-year appropriation, which included a special provision for the restoration of the cosmetics program. The agency has since reinstated the Voluntary Cosmetic Registration Program.[5] But since the safety of our cosmetics and personal care products rests in the fickle hands of Congress, one must be concerned about how long even this minimal level of regulation will last.

Cosmetics have never had a high rating on the national agenda. During the 1930s, Assistant Secretary of Agriculture Rex Tugwell publicized photographs of women disfigured and occasionally blinded because of hair dyes, eyelash dyes, and other dangerous cosmetics, in an effort to upgrade the 1906 Pure Food and Drug Act. Supporting Tugwell's efforts to give teeth to government-regulated consumer protection, Eleanor Roosevelt noted: "Women want to know what they are buying. What is hiding in that closed can? What are women putting on their skin?" But when the Food, Drug, and Cosmetic Bill finally passed in 1938, Tugwell found the watered-down version "disgraceful." There were "no standards, no grades, no penalties for fraud."[6] Not much has changed over the last sixty years.

Why does Congress place so little importance on the safety of cosmetics? One reason is that the skin was always thought to provide an impervious barrier, preventing the absorption of chemicals applied to it. But with the development of transdermal drug delivery, that belief has been overturned. Today, transdermal medications are commonly used to prevent seasickness, treat angina, or introduce hormones as a symptomatic remedy for menopause. In *A Consumer's Dictionary of Cosmetic Ingredients*, author Ruth Winter points out: "It has now been accepted that *all* chemicals penetrate the skin to some extent, and many do so in significant amounts. Good tests for skin penetration are available, yet they are rarely used for cosmetics."[7]

So, just how much of these chemicals are transmitted into the bloodstream through your skin? It depends on how they are introduced. Powders have the least absorption. Oily solutions or those designed to increase moisture allow more of the chemical to be absorbed. The condition of the skin also plays a part. Damaged skin is much more permeable than intact skin, so if you have a cut or a flare-up of acne, your skin is more susceptible to chemical absorption.

Your skin isn't the only way by which toxic chemicals can enter your body. Eye makeup can be absorbed by the highly sensitive mucous membranes. Hair sprays, perfumes, and dusting powders can be inhaled, irritating the lungs. Lipstick is often chewed off and swallowed.

The FDA acknowledges these methods of absorption and strongly urges safety testing before a product is made available to consumers, yet it can't force manufacturers to comply. The FDA can take action regarding the safety of a product only after a problem develops from its use. Even then, the FDA isn't automatically permitted to require the manufacturer to recall the product. Recalls of defective or hazardous products are left to the discretion of the cosmetics company. According to a fact sheet published by the FDA, "If the FDA wishes to remove a cosmetic product from the market, it must first prove in a court of law that the product may be injurious to users, improperly labeled, or otherwise violates the law."[8]

Although the FDA has managed to prohibit a few ingredients that have proved hazardous to human health and the environment (including bithionol, mercury compounds, chloroform, and hexachlorophene[9]), without strict governmental guidelines for ingredients, cosmetics manufacturers can put anything they please into their products. In fact, the laws regulating safety of cosmetics are so weak that during congressional hearings in 1988, then-Representative Wyden commented, "The FDA's existing authority to regulate cosmetics is no better than a toothless pit bull guarding a multimillion-dollar mansion."[10]

While most cosmetics companies voluntarily test their products for common sensitivities, researchers from the National Research Council found that "Of the tens of thousands of commercially important chemicals, only a few have been subjected to extensive toxicity testing and most have scarcely been tested at all."[11] In other words, the mere fact that a product shows up on the market doesn't mean it's safe.

The Legacy of Industrial Science

Of the limited number of cosmetics chemicals that have been tested, many are known to have the potential to cause cancer. Others are suspected carcinogens. But what does that really mean? While we're all far too familiar with the concept of cancer, most of us don't know how years of exposure to certain chemicals can result in this dreaded disease.

Chronic exposure to cancer-causing chemicals can change the way our cells function. Under normal circumstances, our cells behave in predictable ways. If you get a cut, the cells surrounding the wound automatically reproduce to fill in the injured area with new, healthy cells. Once their mission is accomplished, these healthy cells know when to stop reproducing. Sometimes, however, cells are altered and begin reproducing in a disorderly way for no apparent reason, often clustering together to form a malignant lump or tumor. Eventually, this tumor can spread to other parts of the body, interfering with the normal functioning of the body's organs, tissues, and cells. Given the vast number of environmental carcinogens to which we're exposed every day, it's not surprising that cell mutations occur quite frequently. Luckily, the immune system's normal surveillance usually detects and destroys these potentially cancerous cells, effectively eliminating the threat.

Unfortunately, other factors, known as "indirect" carcinogens, can interfere with this search-and-destroy mechanism. Indirect carcinogens actually promote cellular growth by suppressing the immune system or by interfering with the way our hormones function. Some indirect carcinogens, such as dioxin, can also increase the production of certain proteins, activating chemicals that bind to DNA, causing them to mutate.

There are more than a hundred varieties of cancer, each of which has different causes, symptoms, and rates of development. However, most cancers fall into one of four categories. Carcinomas affect the skin, mucous membranes, glands, and internal organs; leukemias are cancers of the blood-forming tissues; lymphomas affect the lymphatic system; and sarcomas target muscles, connective tissue, and bone. Most carcinogens found in cosmetics are considered carcinomas and lymphomas. Cancer is on the rise. Over the past thirty years, the rate of brain and other central nervous system cancers, breast cancer, multiple myeloma, kidney cancer, non-Hodgkin's lymphoma, and melanoma has increased 20 percent.[12] In the United States alone, one person dies from cancer every minute.[13] While some cancers can be linked to hereditary factors, researchers now believe that 85 to 95 percent of today's cancer can be traced to environmental exposure—from the foods we eat, the air we breathe, and the chemicals we use.

Many of these carcinogenic chemicals can be found in everyday cosmetics. Ironically, these products are the foundation of an industry/community-based partnership targeting cancer victims. Under the banner of the American Cancer Society, the "Look Good . . . Feel Better" program was founded and developed by the Cosmetic, Toiletry, and Fragrance Association,[14] the industry bulldog of cosmetics manufacturers. The program is geared toward women undergoing chemotherapy and radiation treatments. Its goal is to help enhance appearance and self-image through the use of conventional cosmetics, once again emphasizing the cosmetics industry's desire to put image before health.

Hormones Gone Haywire

It's no longer just the cancer-causing effects of chemicals about which we need to worry. In the late 1970s, scientists discovered a new threat, one with far-reaching effects that could have an impact not only on our own health but also on the health of our unborn children.

Endocrine disruptors are chemicals that interfere with the normal functioning of the body's hormones by either blocking the body's natural estrogen or acting like an estrogen impostor. Unlike natural estrogens, called phytoestrogens, these synthetic endocrine disruptors accumulate in the body. While natural estrogens are vital to normal human development, synthetic hormone disruptors have been linked to a reduction in sperm, impaired thyroid function, breast cancer, and even behavioral problems such as attention deficit hyperactivity disorder (ADHD).

Although very few cosmetics ingredients have been thoroughly tested for their reproductive or developmental effects, it is believed that a steady stream of exposure to these suspected endocrine-disrupting chemicals can be particularly dangerous for pregnant women, even in low doses. Not only can they affect the unborn fetus, but also some of these ingredients have been found in human breast milk—making them a concern for nursing mothers.[15] Here are a few of the endocrine-disrupting chemicals that may be hiding in your cosmetics:

Dioxins

One recognized endocrine disruptor is dioxin, a term actually referring to a family of seventy-five toxic chlorinated chemicals.[16] Dioxins became prevalent in the environment after World War II as a consequence of the rising production and use of chlorine-based chemicals. Known as the most potent carcinogen ever studied, dioxin in an amount the size of a fist is toxic enough to kill every person on Earth.

Formed as an accidental by-product of many industrial processes, including the creation of plastic and the bleaching of paper, dioxin accumulates in the body's fatty tissue. It can cause chloracne, a disfiguring skin condition that produces skin eruptions, cysts, and pustules. Long-term or prenatal exposure to dioxin can cause birth defects, cardiovascular and nervous system damage, endometriosis, and a variety of cancers, including leukemia and cancer of the breast and prostate.[17]

Are your cosmetics harboring hidden dioxin? Probably, particularly if you use deodorants or antibacterial soaps. Dioxins can also enter our bathrooms in the form of packaging and commercially bleached cotton balls and tissues. Even the plastic bottles we love to collect may contain dioxins that can leach into the shampoos, body washes, and skin creams we use every day.

Alkylphenol Ethoxylates

Another category of endocrine disruptor that may affect the hormonal, neurological, immune, and reproductive systems is alkylphenol ethoxylates. Alkylphenol ethoxylates are a class of surfactants used for their detergent or oil-dispersing properties. One surfactant of particular concern is nonylphenol, an estrogen mimic that can be found in some plastics, as well as shampoos, hair colors, and shaving creams.

Created as a by-product during the breakdown of certain chemicals commonly found in cosmetics, nonylphenols were discovered to be estrogenic quite by accident. In 1987, Boston researchers Ana Soto and Carlos Sonnenschein headed to their laboratory at Tufts University School of Medicine to check on some human breast cell cultures. The cultures had been placed in small cups, along with a blood serum, some of which contained various levels of estrogen. Neither researcher expected anything unusual when they set the cultures under the microscope. But what they found was truly astounding. The breast cells, both those with added estrogen and those without, were multiplying like crazy! After months of detective work, Soto and Sonnenschein discovered the culprit. The plastic test tubes used to store the blood serum had leached an estrogen-like substance into the fluid. Why did these particular test tubes behave differently? The manufacturer had recently added a chemical to make the plastic more stable and less breakable—nonylphenol.[18]

Manufacturers often add nonylphenols to polyvinyl chloride (commonly known as PVC), a common ingredient in nail enamels. But this type of surfactant isn't always a deliberate addition. A by-product of Soto and Sonnenschein's investigation was the discovery that the breakdown of some chemicals found in personal care products can also give rise to nonylphenol.

Nonylphenols are persistent in the environment, making them a health risk that can affect fertility and reproductive development in both men and women. Long-term exposure could also encourage the proliferation of breast and uterine tissue, ultimately leading to a higher risk of developing these cancers. The health and environmental threat is so serious that, in 1992, fourteen European and Scandinavian countries agreed to phase out all alkylphenols by the year 2000.[19]

Parabens

On the outskirts of London, a group of British researchers at Brunel University recently discovered another type of hormone-disrupting chemical—parabens. Although considered safe for use in cosmetics (parabens gained favor with cosmetics manufacturers in the late 1970s because of their broad-spectrum antibacterial properties), the study found that parabens also mimic estrogen.[20] Yet another in vivo study of parabens found they had estrogenic potencies comparable to bisphenol-A.[21]

Usually preceded with the prefixes *methyl-*, *ethyl-*, *propyl-*, or *butyl-*, parabens are potent preservatives that can be found in everything from shampoos to skin creams. "Given their use in a wide range of commercially available topical preparations," noted the authors of the Brunel study, "it is suggested that the safety of these chemicals should now be reassessed."

Phthalates

Phthalates (pronounced "thay-lates") are another type of endocrine disruptor. Used to make plastic soft and pliable, this compound came under attack in late 1998 when Greenpeace issued a report pointing out the danger phthalates pose when used to create soft plastic toys.[22] Since these plasticizers don't bond with the plastic itself, they can easily leach out into saliva or other liquids. Long-term exposure is suspected of causing damage to the kidneys, liver, and reproductive organs.

Although it's believed that phthalate exposure comes mainly from foods that have absorbed the chemical from its plastic packaging, these plasticizers can also be found in your bathroom. Used as ingredients in hair spray, perfume, and nail polishes, phthalates are likely to accumulate in body fat.

Because the effects of these and other synthetic chemicals develop over the course of several decades, it's difficult to find a direct cause-and-effect scenario for certain chemical ingredients. A sixty-year-old woman who develops breast cancer wouldn't even think of blaming the makeup she's used every day for the past forty years. The other problem is that, over the past fifty years, we've been exposed to a variety of toxins in our air, water, and food. It's impossible to pinpoint one specific chemical or product. Researchers can, however, predict possible health risks based on the information currently available. Although not conclusive, this body of data could lead manufacturers in the right direction.

New evidence is constantly being discovered regarding the carcinogenic and endocrine-disrupting properties of synthetic chemicals. Yet, cosmetics companies continue to ignore this potentially health-threatening evidence. It's an attitude of "make a buck today—tomorrow will take care of itself" that could, in the long run, cost consumers their lives. Fortunately, consumers can take some simple steps to minimize the risks of chronic exposure to these harmful synthetic chemicals.

Learn to Read Labels

Buying beauty products at a drugstore or department store can leave your head swimming. If you rely solely on the descriptions located on the front of the package, you're likely to be misled. Manufacturers of shampoos, bath preparations, and makeup bandy around words such as *natural, botanical,* and *organic.* But what do all those comforting words really mean? Not much, according to most consumer advocates. There are no legal definitions when it comes to cosmetics, only creative advertising copy designed to give shoppers a "feeling" for the product instead of giving them the information they need.

In response to growing consumer interest, manufacturers have jumped on the term *natural,* making it the most abused word in marketing. But buyer, beware. According to John Bailey, director of the FDA's Office of Cosmetics and Colors: "There are no standards for what natural means. They [the manufacturers] could wave a tube of plant extract over a bottle and declare it natural."[23] Since many of today's cosmetics and personal care products contain some natural ingredients, manufacturers may be technically correct in touting a product as natural or botanical, even if the bulk of ingredients comes from a chemist's lab. But a dab of aloe vera or a sprinkling of herbs doesn't mean the product is chemical-free.

As far as cosmetics are concerned, the term *organic* doesn't fare much better. Unlike organic foods, which are currently regulated under some state guidelines, cosmetics have no standards to adhere to. In an effort to remedy this lack of regulation, Aubrey Organics, a natural cosmetics manufacturer, has filed a citizen petition with the FDA to extend organic food guidelines to include skin and hair care.[24]

What about hypoallergenic cosmetics? In 1975, the FDA tried to publish regulations defining *hypoallergenic* as having a lower potential for allergic reactions but succeeded only in raising the industry's ire. Almay and Clinique objected to the proposed regulation, claiming the public knew that, even though a product was labeled hypoallergenic, allergic reactions were still possible. The courts agreed, essentially leaving cosmetics manufacturers in control of defining products in any way they see fit.[25]

The best way to protect yourself from the cosmetics industry's dance with semantics is to learn to read ingredient labels. To get you started, let's look at the ingredients of a popular off-the-shelf shampoo that touts a botanical blend supposedly designed to protect hair against moisture loss:

CONTAINS: Purified Water, Ammonium Lauryl Sulfate, Ammonium Laureth Sulfate, Glycerin, Lauramide DEA, Honeydew Melon Juice, Rose Oil, Methenamine, Honey Extract, Nettle Extract, Hydroxy-

propyl Methylcellulose, Tetrasodium EDTA, Ammonium Chloride,
Panthenol, Sodium PCA, Cocamidopropyl Hydroxysultaine, Cetyl
Palmitate, Dipropylene Glycol, DMDM Hydantoin, Ammonium
Xylensulfonate, Citric Acid, Propylene Glycol, Fragrance, Sodium
Lauryl Sulfate, Cocamide-DEA, Glycol Stearate, PEG-60 Hydro-
genated Castor Oil, D&C Red No. 33, FD&C Yellow No. 5

The ingredients are listed in descending order, with the largest amount
of a particular ingredient listed first. Of the twenty-nine ingredients in this
particular product, most are synthetic and many are petroleum based. Besides
having difficulty pronouncing them, the average shopper has no idea what
they are or how they might impact the buyer's health. Only five are easily identified as natural—purified water, honeydew melon, rose oil, and honey and
nettle extracts. But nothing on the label tells consumers how much of these
natural substances are used and at what strength.

Take a closer look at what you're really buying:

Ammonium Lauryl Sulfate is a mild surfactant cleanser.
Ammonium Laureth Sulfate is a compound that breaks up and holds oil.
　　Both these chemicals are mild irritants.
Glycerin is a solvent, humectant, and emollient. The FDA issued a notice
　　in 1992 that glycerin has not been shown to be safe or effective.
Lauramide DEA is used as a softener and foam inhibitor. It may be con-
　　taminated with nitrosamines.
Methenamine is made from formaldehyde and ammonia. It is one of the
　　most frequent causes of skin irritation.
Hydroxypropyl Methylcellulose is used as an emulsifier.
Tetrasodium EDTA, a chelating agent, is an eye and skin irritant.
Ammonium Chloride is used as an acidifier. If ingested, it can cause nau-
　　sea, vomiting, and acidosis.
Panthenol is a vitamin B complex and is actually good for the scalp.
Sodium PCA, a naturally occurring component of human skin, is used
　　to soften hair. The synthetic version can dry skin and cause severe
　　allergic reactions.
Cocamidopropyl Hydroxysultaine is a synthetic derivative of coconut
　　oil and is used as a secondary surfactant.
Cetyl Palmitate is produced by the reaction of cetyl alcohol and palmitic
　　acid.

Dipropylene Glycol is used as a solvent and wetting agent and is related to propylene glycol.

DMDM Hydantoin is a toxic compound used as a preservative and contains 17.7 percent formaldehyde.

Ammonium Xylensulfonate is a solvent often used in nail polish. Chronic toxicity is not known.

Citric Acid is used widely in cosmetics as a preservative, foam inhibitor, and plasticizer and to adjust the acid-alkali balance.

Propylene Glycol is a moisture-carrying vehicle. The safety of this neurotoxin is questionable.

Fragrance could be either natural or synthetic. It is the leading cause of allergic reactions from cosmetics use and may be carcinogenic.

Sodium Lauryl Sulfate is used as a wetting agent, detergent, and emulsifier. With the potential to form nitrosamines, it can irritate and dry the skin.

Cocamide-DEA is a hair conditioner, surfactant, and thickener and may be contaminated by nitrosamines.

Glycol Stearate is one of the most widely used bases for cosmetics even though it can cause allergic reactions.

PEG-60 Hydrogenated Castor Oil is a plasticizing agent and solvent that has been shown to cause cancer in laboratory animals.

D&C Red No. 33 is a coloring agent. The FDA is currently investigating complex scientific and legal questions regarding this substance.

FD&C Yellow No. 5 is a coal tar derivative that may cause allergic reactions in people sensitive to aspirin.[26]

Nine Deadly Ingredients

Overwhelmed? It's not surprising. There are more than fifty-five hundred cosmetics ingredients approved for use by the FDA.[27] Although not all of these chemicals undermine your health, the National Institute of Occupational Safety and Health reports that 884 of the ingredients used in cosmetics are toxic.[28] Here are facts on nine of the worst offenders:

1. **Coal tar colors** are made from the liquid or semisolid tar found in bituminous coal and can contain a number of toxins such as benzene, xylene, naphthalene, phenol, and creosol. Coal tar is poisonous in its pure state, and

almost all of these colors have been shown to cause cancer, making their use highly controversial. Adding to this controversy is the problem of sensitivity. Coal tar is a phototoxin, and many people experience allergic reactions when exposed to products containing coal tar derivatives.[29]

All FD&C and D&C colors are made from coal tar, yet most have never been tested for safety. They were grandfathered into the cosmetics industry's repertoire under the 1938 Federal Food, Drug, and Cosmetic Act, and the World Health Organization considers them probable carcinogens.[30] Public Citizen, a consumer advocacy group founded by Ralph Nader, has also questioned the safety of coal tar colors and considers them all unsafe.[31]

Even though the FDA maintains that the risk of cancer from coal tar colors is minimal, a provisional listing of these untested colors was compiled by the agency in 1960. Colors on this "temporary" list were allowed to be used in cosmetics until safety studies had been completed and each color was either placed on the permanent GRAS (Generally Recognized As Safe) list or else banned from use. The original intention was to abolish the provisional list once the safety of its contents had been determined. However, only a handful of colors have been tested for safety, and the bulk of colors remain on the list thirty years later.[32]

Even colors that at one time were believed safe and placed on the GRAS list can be removed if found to be hazardous. FD&C Orange Nos. 1 and 2 and FD&C Red No. 32 were banned in 1950 after children were made ill from their use in candy and popcorn. More recently, FD&C colors Red No. 1, Violet No. 1, and Yellow Nos. 1 through 4 were taken off the list. In 1976, Red No. 2, the most widely used FD&C color, was banned because it caused tumors in rats. That same year, Red No. 4 and carbon black were found to be carcinogenic and were removed from the list. Unless a color additive receives a lot of publicity, as was the case with Red No. 2, most consumers are unaware of the impact that long-term use of coal tar colors can have on their health.

Although all coal tar colors are potentially carcinogenic, there are several of which to be especially wary when you are choosing a product. *Anthraquinone* dyes, which include Ext. D&C Violet No. 2, are a particularly nasty family of dyes made from phthalic anhydride and benzene. They may cause skin irritation, allergic reactions, and contact dermatitis. They have also been found to cause tumors in laboratory animals.[33] *Azo* dyes, used in nonpermanent hair rinses and tints, are absorbed through the skin and can cause allergic reactions.[34] *Quinoline* is created when coal tar interacts with aniline, acetaldehyde, and formaldehyde—all extremely toxic and carcinogenic. D&C

Yellow Nos. 10 and 11, as well as other artificial colors often found in dandruff shampoos, are from the quinoline family.[35] Made from carbon tetrachloride, benzene, and aluminum chloride, *triphenylmethane* dyes are highly carcinogenic. Included among the dyes in this group are FD&C Blue No. 1 and FD&C Green Nos. 1 through 3.[36] *Xanthenes* are colorants used most often in lipsticks. They can be found under the names FD&C Red No. 3 and D&C Red Nos. 2 and 19 and may cause phototoxicity.[37]

Since coal tar colors are used so extensively in cosmetics, it's a good idea to search out products containing natural coloring agents. Natural alternatives such as annatto, beta-carotene, and henna are derived from plants and have been safely used for centuries.

2. Formaldehyde can be found in nail polish, nail hardeners, soap, shampoos, and hair growth preparations. Hydantoins and surfactants, such as sodium lauryl sulfate, may contain formaldehyde even when it's not listed on the label. An economical and effective preservative, it's also widely used in cosmetics as a disinfectant, germicide, fungicide, and defoamer.

Since formaldehyde is a naturally occurring chemical found within the human body in minute amounts, the Formaldehyde Institute claims this chemical is part of the normal life process. Yet, it is estimated that 20 percent of people exposed to this noxious chemical develop a toxic reaction.[38] Studies have also shown it to cause lung cancer in laboratory tests, and it's been found to damage DNA. In light of these studies, the National Cancer Institute's Division of Cancer Cause and Prevention has recommended further investigation into formaldehyde's effect on human health.[39]

The FDA had, at one time, banned the use of formaldehyde but has since allowed it to be used in limited concentrations. Although it is outlawed in Sweden and Japan, the European Economic Community also allows its use but only if concentrations of 0.05 percent or greater are listed on the product label.[40] Unfortunately, this label requirement isn't deemed necessary by the government of the United States.

3. Lead, in any form, is poisonous. Yet, it can be found in some hair dyes, especially those that work gradually. Although the FDA approved the use of lead acetate in progressive hair dyes in 1980, it is a known carcinogen and hormone disruptor. Readily absorbed through the skin, lead accumulates in the bones and can be released months or even years later.[41]

A study by Xavier University of Louisiana found a number of brands of hair dyes that contain up to ten times the amount of lead allowed in household paint. Howard Mielke, the toxicologist who presented the study, found that, after dying his own hair, there was lead contamination on the hair dryer, the sink, and his skin—so much that it couldn't be washed off his hands![42]

The toxicity of lead is cumulative, building up in the body over the course of many years, and its effects can be severe. There is strong evidence that lead exposure can also cause subtle neurological damage and behavioral abnormalities.[43] Leg cramps, muscle weakness, numbness, depression, brain damage, and coma can result from large accumulations of this toxic metal.

Because exposure to lead poses such an extreme threat to human health, the Center for Environmental Health recently filed a lawsuit against Combe, Inc., the manufacturer of the Grecian Formula line, under California's Proposition 65.[44] Proposition 65 requires that manufacturers include warning labels on products that exceed safety standards.

4. Nitrosamines, though not a primary ingredient in cosmetics, are also cautionary chemicals. Nitrosamines are formed when two otherwise safe chemicals, nitrous acid and amines, are combined. The resulting carcinogen can contaminate shampoo or other products where this chemical reaction occurs. Nitrosamine contamination can occur during the storage of raw materials or when a product is processed. According to a 1978 FDA report, shampooing with a product containing nitrosamines can lead to its absorption into the body at levels higher than eating a nitrate-contaminated food.[45]

A number of nitrosating agents are commonly used in cosmetics, including diethanolamine (DEA), triethanolamine (TEA), monoethanolamine (MEA), formaldehyde, and sodium lauryl (or laureth) sulfate. These ingredients are often combined with other synthetic chemicals—for example, cocamide-DEA or TEA lauryl sulfate. To be on the safe side, consumer advocates recommend avoiding all products that contain DEA, TEA, or MEA compounds.

5. Phenylenediamine, often preceded by m-, o-, or p-, is found in permanent hair dyes, commonly known as oxidation dyes or peroxide dyes. Protected under the 1938 FDA exemption, phenylenediamine can adversely react with other chemicals and result in photosensitivity. Phenylenediamine can also cause eczema, bronchial asthma, gastritis, skin irritations, and even death. Although the FDA is unable to ban its use, the agency proposed a requirement ordering manufacturers to place warning labels on products containing this substance. If the proposal were accepted, the label would have read, "Warning: [this product] contains an ingredient that can penetrate your skin and has been determined to cause cancer in laboratory animals." At the same time, the FDA also proposed that beauty salons using these products post warnings for their customers. Cosmetics industry lobbyists successfully defeated both proposals, and no warnings were ever seen on products containing phenylenediamine.[46]

6. **Propylene Glycol**, an ingredient used in antifreeze and brake fluid, is also used as a delivery vehicle and solvent in place of glycerin. Cheaper and more readily absorbed than glycerin, propylene glycol is found in numerous beauty preparations. In fact, it's the most widely used moisture-carrying ingredient found in cosmetics. This chemical is acknowledged as a neurotoxin by the National Institute for Occupational Safety and Health,[47] and recent studies have tied it to contact dermatitis, kidney damage, and liver abnormalities.[48] It also inhibits skin cell growth, directly altering cell membranes.

When drums of propylene glycol are delivered to cosmetics manufacturers by suppliers, the Material Safety Data Sheet required to accompany the shipment explicitly warns workers to "Avoid skin contact."[49] Why, then, is this ingredient still being used in everything from baby lotions to mascara?

7. **Quaternary Ammonium Compounds** are used as preservatives, surfactants, and germicides in a wide range of cosmetics. All quaternary compounds can be toxic, depending on the concentration and dose. Often listed on ingredient labels as benzalkonium chloride, cetrimonium bromide, and quaternium 1-29, quaternary ammonium compounds are caustic and can irritate the skin and eyes.

Originally used as a fabric softener, these compounds can make hair and skin feel softer immediately after use. But in the long run, repeated use will sap moisture from the skin cells, leaving hair and skin dry and flaky.

Of all the quaternary ammonium compounds to avoid, benzalkonium chloride is the most toxic. Because of its high toxicity, the FDA proposed banning the use of benzalkonium chloride in over-the-counter insect remedies and astringent drugs in 1992.[50] Quaternium-15, another cautionary ingredient, is a formaldehyde releaser and, according to the American Academy of Dermatology, is the number one cause of preservative-related contact dermatitis.[51]

8. Sodium Lauryl Sulfate is found in 90 percent of all commercial shampoos, as well as skin creams and some toothpastes. Popular with cosmetics manufacturers because of its lathering properties, sodium lauryl sulfate is a known skin irritant. According to a report published in *The Lancet*, sodium lauryl sulfate damages the skin barrier function, enhancing the allergic response to other toxins and allergens, as well as altering skin cells.[52] What's more, the FDA recently warned cosmetics manufacturers of unacceptable levels of dioxin formation in some products containing sodium lauryl sulfate.[53]

This ingredient can also react with other chemicals to form nitrosamines. Whether or not a particular bottle of shampoo or jar of skin cream is contaminated with these toxins can be determined only through laboratory testing.

9. Talc is an ingredient that, on the surface, seems relatively benign. After all, what feels better on a hot summer's eve than a cool dusting of fragrant talcum powder? But underneath that silky smooth feeling lies a potentially deadly substance. According to studies by the Occupational Safety and Health Administration, talc is carcinogenic in animals.[54] Further studies conducted by Linda Cook, M.D., of the Fred Hutchinson Cancer Research Center in Seattle, found that women who regularly use talc in the genital area increase their risk of developing ovarian cancer threefold. Chemically similar to asbestos, talc-based products migrate up the vaginal canal to the reproductive tract.[55]

Airborne talc particles can also be a hazard. The talc in body powders and antiperspirant sprays can irritate the lungs when inhaled. And since talcum powder has been reported to cause coughing, vomiting, and even pneumonia by some users, pediatricians are now warning new parents to avoid using talc-based products on their children.

Talc can also be found in blushes, eye shadows, face powders, liquid foundations, and even skin fresheners. Although it gives products a slippery feel, talc used near the eyes can irritate sensitive mucous membranes.

Inert Doesn't Mean Harmless

The most confusing ingredients found in cosmetics and personal care products are the "inert" elements. Inert ingredients don't make the product work. They are often used to make a product last longer before spoiling or as a processing agent to make the finished result more spreadable, more sprayable, or less concentrated, or to add a nice color or fragrance.

Inert ingredients have received little attention, mainly because most of us consider them innocent additives. Yet, artificial colors and fragrances are a frequent cause of allergic reactions and can contain carcinogenic elements. Emulsifiers, including potassium and sodium stearates, polysorbates, poloxamers, and surfactants, can dry skin and cause irritation and inflammation.

Since most cosmetics are made in large batches and can sit on store shelves for months, strong preservatives are required to keep the ingredients from separating and to protect them from microbial, bacterial, and fungal contamination. The most commonly used preservatives are methyl- and propylparabens, endocrine disruptors that are strong sensitizers, and DMDM hydantoin, which may release formaldehyde. Another highly used preservative found in nearly all cosmetics preparations is imidazolidinyl urea. According to the American Academy of Dermatology, it is found to cause contact dermatitis.[56]

Chemical Cocktails

We've seen the risks of a number of individual chemicals, but what happens when these isolated substances are combined? Studies have shown that even relatively safe chemicals can interact when combined with each other, creating new, and possibly unsafe, chemicals. It's unrealistic to assume that each chemical acts independently of other chemicals in the same product, yet that's just what current government regulation and toxicology testing methods do. Even though modern cosmetics are an intricate mix of a variety of chemicals, current laws ignore the possibility of interactive effects. As we've seen with nitrosamines, even two harmless ingredients can create a toxin when combined.

Although exposure to a single toxin may be well tolerated by the body, complex combinations of synthetic chemicals may be unsafe.[57] Until the FDA and industry toxicologists begin addressing this concern, consumers have no way to assess the risks of these chemical cocktails.

Sense and Sensitivities

Cosmetics manufacturers routinely test for common sensitivities. It may seem like a minor concern in comparison with the looming threats of long-term cosmetics use, but to the 20 percent of the population who suffer from sensitivities to the chemicals frequently found in cosmetics, it's anything but minor. In fact, it's estimated that, in a single year, more than 200,000 visits to the emergency room are related to allergic reactions from cosmetics use.[58]

Sherrie Solheim Nattrass's skin had always been sensitive, especially to petrochemical products. It was one of the main reasons she had started her own natural cosmetics company. Sherrie believed in using only pure, petrochemical-free ingredients in her products and often tested new cosmetics on herself with no adverse reactions—until a testing session in 1993. Immediately after she used a newly developed vitamin E–based skin cream, her face and neck became swollen and red. Tiny, painful bumps covered the entire area where the cream had been applied. Within the next few days, her eyes had swollen shut and she suffered bouts of weakness and dizziness. Terrified, she rushed to the doctor, who diagnosed a contact reaction to something contained in the skin cream. For the life of her, Sherrie couldn't understand what had caused this acute reaction. Although she knew that the skin cream suspected of causing her illness contained high levels of vitamin E, the substance had never bothered her. After a little research, she found that the chemist had substituted a synthetic form of vitamin E—one derived from petrochemical sources.

The manufacturer had assured the chemist that there was virtually no difference between the synthetic vitamin E he was peddling and the real thing. But in 1996, the FDA confirmed that the artificial version, listed on many products as tocopherol, is completely different from naturally occurring vitamin E.[59] As Sherrie discovered, even ingredients that sound natural can be synthetically derived.

The development of chemical sensitivities can occur at any time, even if you've used a particular product for years. Perhaps the manufacturer changed the formula. Or you may be taking a medication that creates a hypersensitivity. Age can be another factor. Normally, the younger you are, the less tolerance you may have for certain chemicals. A twelve- or thirteen-year-old girl just starting to use makeup may not be able to tolerate the same amount of a chemical substance that a forty-year-old woman could. But just because you've passed puberty, don't assume you're safe from chemical sensitivities. Adults can suddenly develop adverse reactions to familiar products since, as we age, we accumulate increasing levels of environmental toxins that can impair our natural resistance to some chemicals. Stress, illness, even hormonal changes such as pregnancy or menopause can also trigger the onset of chemical sensitivity.

If you do have an adverse reaction to a cosmetic or personal care product, stop using it. If the reaction is severe, see a doctor immediately and discuss possible chemical causes for your symptoms. If you can pinpoint which product caused the problem, notify the manufacturer and the FDA. A listing for your local FDA office should appear in your telephone book under "U.S. Government."

There are precautions you can take if you suffer from long-term sensitivities. Read the ingredient label before buying any cosmetic. If you're not sure whether a specific allergen or sensitizer is included in a particular product, contact the manufacturer before using it. If you know you're prone to chemical sensitivities, do a skin test before using any new product. Simply apply a small amount of the product to your forearm and check the area after twenty-four hours. If you see any redness or skin irritation, or if you experience burning or itching, don't use the product.

A Healthy Deception

So, where can consumers find healthful cosmetics? A number of natural beauty gurus urge consumers to shop at their local health food stores for cosmetics and personal care products. But the fact that a product shares shelf space with natural supplements and organic food doesn't necessarily guarantee that it's chemical-free. Some so-called natural products contain synthetic petrochemicals, especially color cosmetics and hair care products. One such product, a shampoo found at a very reputable health food store, boasted 20 percent natural henna. It also claimed to be biodegradable and cruelty-free. It sounded like a good product. But a closer look revealed a disturbing number of synthetic and potentially harmful chemicals such as lauramide DEA; TEA lauryl sulfate; and germall, a toxic antibacterial.

Although many of these products contain fewer chemical ingredients than their mainstream counterparts, they may still include harmful compounds. Powders, creams, and foundations can contain talc or propylene glycol. Many "natural" shampoos list sodium lauryl sulfate and DEA, MEA, or TEA, all of which can cause the formation of nitrosamines. Benzophenones, which can produce hives or other photoallergic reactions, can be found in hair conditioners, sunscreens, and soaps. Before you purchase any product claiming to be pure, natural, or organic, read the ingredient label to make sure the claims are justified.

Fortunately, a number of responsible companies manufacture truly natural cosmetics without resorting to toxic synthetic chemicals. These cosmetics, too, can be found in health food stores, often sitting right next to a chemically packed version of the same product.

Part II

Natural Alternatives to Chemical Beauty

3

The Alchemist's Secret

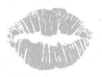

*"Alchemy: The power or process of transforming something
common into something special."*
—*Webster's Dictionary*

As we've become more concerned with the wholesomeness and purity of the beauty products we buy, we've begun taking a serious look at the dozens of natural cosmetics introduced into health food stores every year. Once an obscure market, natural cosmetics are now gaining a strong foothold among mainstream consumers. Yet, while there are a number of quality cosmetics on the market, as we've seen, some products claiming to be "all natural" are anything but.

One way to assure the products you use are pure and natural is to make them yourself. Just as effective as the store-bought varieties, homemade cosmetics cost a small fraction of what you'd pay at the health food store or cosmetics counter. Instead of spending a fortune on high-priced jars of chemicals that might have been sitting on the store shelf for months, you will have fresh, natural products using herbs, grains, fruits, and vegetables.

A word of warning before you begin: while most of us consider synthetic-free cosmetics harmless, there is no such thing as a beauty product that is safe for everyone. If you have a history of allergies, do a skin test before you use any new product, even if you make it yourself. Apply a small amount of the mixture on the inside of your arm and wait twenty-four to forty-eight hours. If you experience a rash, swelling, itching, or redness, don't use the product.

While making your own cosmetics is a simple art to master, you'll need to follow a few general guidelines:

Use Only the Best

It stands to reason that the best homemade cosmetics are those made with the best ingredients. Fresh, high-quality raw materials are the key to success. While it would be ideal if we could walk out to the garden and pluck fresh, perfectly ripe fruits and vegetables or dew-kissed herbs to use in our creams and lotions, for many of us, this isn't an option. Luckily, organic produce and fresh herbs are available in many health food stores and supermarkets. If you opt for store-bought ingredients, choose the freshest items you can find, preferably at their peak of ripeness. Make sure they aren't past their prime— as produce begins to deteriorate, it loses some of its healing properties.

Using fresh herbs can be costly, and some varieties are difficult to find. An alternative is to buy high-quality dried herbs. Although not as potent as their fresh counterparts, properly dried herbs can be an effective substitute. An added bonus is that dried herbs may be stored in a cool, dark spot for a year or more, making it easy to keep an ample supply on hand.

One way to find a wide variety of dried herbs is by using a reputable herb dealer. As the ancient art of herbalism becomes a popular alternative to conventional medicine, herbs are becoming more readily available. Commercial sources often offer herbs in a variety of forms, including whole, cut, and powdered. Although most dealers offer high-quality products, some may use lower-quality herbs or cut their herbs with cheaper, inferior plants. When you receive your order, check the color and aroma of the herbs. High-quality herbs should not appear brown or faded and should have a strong, pungent smell. To find an herb dealer in your area, look in the yellow pages of your local telephone book under the heading "Herbs." If you're not lucky enough to locate an herb dealer nearby, a number of companies will be happy to send you their product catalogs. Check botanical magazines or the listings in the back of this book for dealers offering mail-order services.

Essential oils can also be bought from herb dealers or found in health food and New Age stores. A wonderful addition to cosmetics and aromatherapy preparations, essential oils are the volatile oils produced from herbs, barks, and flowers and contain therapeutic properties that can promote health and well-being. Considered by some to be the spirit of the plant, essential oils are extracted through a process of steam distillation or solvent extraction. To derive the full benefit from essential oils, make sure you purchase a pure product. A good rule of thumb when buying essential oils is that you get what you pay for. Adulterated and synthetic oils have become more prevalent as aromatherapy gains popularity. These products are usually sold at a substantially lower price. True essential oils, although more expensive, will contain the healing properties or, as some aromatherapists believe, the "life force" of the plant itself.

Except for some of the ingredients, you won't have to purchase any special equipment to create your exclusive line of cosmetics. Bowls, saucepans, bottles, jars, measuring cups and spoons, and perhaps a blender are all that you'll need. Do use equipment made of glass or a nonreactive metal such as stainless steel to prevent unexpected chemical reactions. If you plan on using essential oils in your preparations, invest in an inexpensive eyedropper. When you are ready to begin making your own cosmetics, make sure that all of your equipment is scrupulously clean—invisible organisms left on your equipment can quickly spoil a whole batch of cosmetics.

A Glossary of Uncommon Ingredients

Knowing exactly what ingredients you are using and the properties each ingredient possesses will help you create products specifically designed for your skin and hair type. While most of the ingredients you'll be using are familiar—oatmeal, avocados, fruits such as peaches and strawberries—some may not be. Here are some of the more unusual terms and ingredients you may encounter:

Agar
Extracted from various seaweeds, agar is used as an emulsifier and emollient in cosmetics, as well as a substitute for gelatin in foods. Look for it in your health food store.

Aloe Vera
This yellowish, sticky substance is found in the leaves of the aloe vera plant. Noted for healing wounds and burns, aloe vera also soothes and moisturizes skin. Readily available in both gel and liquid form, aloe vera can be found in health food and specialty stores.

Alpha Hydroxy Acids
Appearing naturally in fruits such as coconuts, apples, citrus fruits, and black currants, alpha hydroxy acids, or AHAs, exfoliate and moisturize the skin.

High in glycolic acid, alpha hydroxies have become a popular ingredient among cosmetics manufacturers, which regularly include synthetic AHAs in wrinkle creams, masks, and toners.

Antioxidants

These substances have received a lot of press lately, mainly because of their ability to counteract the destructive effects of free radicals in the body. The most common use of antioxidants, however, is as a preservative. Synthetic antioxidants such as BHA and BHT are often included by cosmetics manufacturers to keep their products from spoiling, but natural antioxidants such as vitamins A, C, and E can be added to cosmetics as safer alternatives to the synthetic variety.

Aromatic Waters

These scented waters are used to treat a variety of skin ailments, from acne to burns. A by-product of distilling essential oils, the most common aromatic water is the familiar rose water. Aromatic waters are expensive and difficult to find. Rose and orange waters are often carried by Indian markets and liquor stores, but these are usually of inferior quality.

Beeswax

Primarily used as an emulsifier, beeswax is obtained from the honeycomb of virgin bees. Because it is insoluble in water, beeswax is a great addition to skin creams and lip balms. For the highest-quality beeswax, purchase it directly from a beekeeper.

Bentonite Clay

This white, moisture-absorbing clay is found in the midwestern United States and is sometimes called Indian Healing Clay. Used in blemish masks, bentonite is reported to draw poisons and toxins out of the skin. It is carried by most health food stores and some drugstores.

Carrier Oils

Vegetable oils are used to dilute and distribute or "carry" a plant's essential oils. Although essential oils don't spoil, some vegetable oils do. To ensure quality, add a bit of vitamin E to your blends as a natural preservative. Commonly used carrier oils include almond, avocado, grape seed, hazelnut, jojoba, olive, and sesame oils.

Castile Soap
Originally made from olive oil, "castile soap" now refers to any mild soap. Although modern castile soaps are widely available, they can be very alkaline to the skin and hair.

Cocoa Butter
Known for its delicious chocolaty aroma, this fat expressed from the roasted seeds of the cocoa plant softens and lubricates the skin. Often used in sun, skin, and massage creams, it melts to an oily consistency.

Cornflower or Corn Flour
An ingredient often listed in British and Australian cosmetics formulas, corn-flower is simply another name for ordinary cornstarch.

Exfoliators
This term refers to any ingredient that promotes the removal of dead skin cells. Natural exfoliators include oatmeal, cornmeal, and almond meal.

Glycerin
A sweet, syrupy by-product of soap making, glycerin has been used for thousands of years as a humectant, emollient, and lubricant in skin care preparations. It is available at most pharmacies.

Henna
This ancient dye comes from the henna shrub and has been used for centuries to color and condition hair. True henna produces a red dye, but today's henna products are mixed with other natural ingredients such as indigo or coffee to produce a variety of shades. Unlike chemical dyes, which penetrate the hair shaft, henna wraps around each strand, effectively sealing it with a reflective coating. It is nontoxic.

Indigo
One of the oldest known nontoxic dyes, indigo is prepared from several plants native to Bengal, Java, and Guatemala. Producing a dark blue powder with

coppery overtones, indigo has been used for centuries to create color cosmetics and hair dye.

Kaolin Clay
Also known as china clay, this fine white mineral clay is used in the manufacture of many powdered and opaque cosmetics. It can also be used as an oil-absorbing face mask. Kaolin clay is more difficult to find than bentonite clay.

Kohl
Used by the Egyptians to line the eye, kohl is reputed to protect the wearer from disease and evil spirits. Originally made from the ash of frankincense, kohl was later made from powdered antimony, a metallic element often containing lead, arsenic, phosphates, and other impurities. Kohls containing lead have been banned in the United States and Great Britain.[1]

Lecithin
This naturally occurring antioxidant and emollient is often used in soaps, skin creams, and hair preparations. Found in egg yolk and soy oil, lecithin is high in the B vitamins choline and inositol. Liquid lecithin is sold in most health food stores.

Orrisroot
Commonly available in craft shops, powdered orrisroot is used in sachets, aromatic dusting powders, and dry shampoos. Derived from the rootstock of the Florentine iris, orris is also used as a fixative in homemade potpourri.

Royal Jelly
Rumored as having the ability to restore the skin's youthfulness, royal jelly is the highly nutritious substance secreted in the throats of worker bees. A valuable component in Chinese medicine, royal jelly contains a full range of amino acids, minerals, enzymes, and vitamins A, B, C, and E. Look for it in Chinese herb shops.

Silica
Critical in the development of strong nails as well as healthy skin and hair, silica is found abundantly in nature. Alfalfa, beets, soybeans, whole grains,

green leafy vegetables, and the herb horsetail are good sources of this important mineral.

Soapwort

A perennial herb used widely during the Middle Ages, soapwort is so-called because the leaves form a lather when bruised. Check with herb dealers for availability.

Tannic Acid

Natural tannic acid can be found in the bark of oak trees as well as in cherries, tea, and coffee. Used as an astringent, tannic acid may tint the hair and skin brown when applied topically.

Volatile Oils

Another name for essential oils, volatile oils are responsible for producing the aroma in certain plants and flowers. Volatile oils stimulate the tissue with which they come in contact and can arouse or soothe, depending on their source and concentration.

Witch Hazel

Used in many synthetic and natural cosmetic preparations, witch hazel is valued for its astringent properties. An old Native American remedy for insect bites, burns, and irritated skin, witch hazel tones the skin and is good for oily complexions. It is available at health food stores and drugstores.

Nature's Technology

You've gathered your equipment and bought your ingredients . . . now what? How do you turn that fragrant rosemary into a body-building hair rinse or those luscious avocados into a moisturizing mask? The methods described in this section will help you turn your raw ingredients into usable cosmetics.

Teas

Making a tea is one of the simplest ways to prepare herbs, flowers, barks, spices, and nuts. While tea is traditionally drunk as a beverage, cosmetics teas are used alone or in combination with other natural ingredients to form a variety of beauty preparations. There are several methods used to prepare cosmetics teas:

Infusions are made much the way you would make a cup of tea. Used to extract the active ingredients from delicate herbs and flowers, infusions prevent the loss of volatile elements often destroyed by prolonged exposure to heat. To make an infusion, pour boiling water over the herbs or flowers. Cover the pan or bowl to retain the plant's essential oils, and steep for 5 to 10 minutes. Strain the tea, cool, and use as is or in your favorite recipe.

Decoctions are used to extract the properties and color from roots, barks, and seeds. To prepare, boil the plant parts in water over high heat for 15 to 30 minutes. The high heat releases more of the active properties from these botanicals than simmering. Strain out the plant material, and cool before using.

Cold infusions use cold water to extract the properties from especially delicate and fragrant herbs and flowers. To make a cold infusion, add about twice the amount of plant material you would use for a normal infusion to a nonmetallic pot of cold water. Cover and steep for 8 to 12 hours before straining.

Vinegars

Although not as potent as teas, herbal vinegars make wonderful hair rinses and skin washes. To make an herbal vinegar, select about 4 ounces of the herb of your choice and place it in a wide-mouth jar. Cover the herb with apple cider vinegar, leaving 2 inches of headroom at the top. Cap and let stand in a cool place, shaking gently once or twice a day. After two weeks, strain, and pour the vinegar into a decorative bottle.

Compresses

A compress is simply a clean cloth or towel soaked in an infusion or decoction and then wrung out and applied to the skin. Compresses can be used either hot or cold, depending on the application, and are a wonderful addition to a home facial. To open clogged pores and dislodge impurities, try a hot (not scalding) compress. A cold compress will tighten pores and stimulate circulation.

Body Oils

A beautiful bottle of heavenly aromatic oil used for bath and massage can fetch a hefty price. Make your own scented body oils by combining 1 ounce of fresh or dried herbs with a pint of carrier oil. Heat to 80°F for several hours (or set it out in the sun on a warm day), and then strain into a decorative bottle. To make a fragrant body oil using essential oils, simply combine a quart of vegetable oil with 4 to 8 drops of your favorite essential oil. Let stand for two weeks, shaking daily to distribute the essential oil.

Purees

If you plan on making lotions and balms, learning to puree is essential. This method is usually reserved for fruits and some vegetables. You may want to use an electric blender to ensure a smooth texture. Peel, pit, and cut your produce into uniform pieces. Toss into the blender and process until smooth.

Sachets and Bath Bags

Lending a romantic touch to your boudoir, sachets and bath bags are a snap to make. Simply cut a 3-inch square of fabric, and fill it with one or more fragrant herbs or flowers. For sachets, choose a pretty velvet or satin, and secure it with a decorative ribbon. Tuck sachets into clothing drawers to keep garments fresh and aromatic. For bath bags, use cheesecloth. Close the top with a piece of long string or ribbon, and suspend the bag under the tap as you fill the tub.

Armed with these simple methods, you will be able to create a variety of fresh, natural skin and hair care products. To get started, check the end of the next several chapters for formulas you can use to create your own natural cosmetics. Think of these formulas as a starting point. As you become more comfortable making your own beauty products, you may want to experiment with various ingredients to create cosmetics that are yours alone.

4

About Face: Skin Care

"A good face is the best letter of recommendation."
—Queen Elizabeth I

Our face is the canvas upon which we write our life stories . . . every line, every expression has its own tale to tell. The emotions that play across our faces connect us to one another. It's the first thing people notice about us. No wonder we place so much importance on the appearance of our faces.

Yet, over the past fifty years, the face has been trivialized. Madison Avenue has created a look that the Western world has come to regard as gospel—classic bones, flawless skin, and, most important, youth. It's a standard to which very few of us can live up—harder still as we age. Yet, we do everything in our power—and our pocketbooks—to achieve and maintain this fantasy of "perfection." We'll spend a king's ransom on chemically packed blemish formulas, wrinkle creams infused with vitamins and hormones, and, in some cases, even major surgery so that we can "face the world." Perhaps it's time to stop chasing someone else's rainbow and take a realistic look in the mirror. While there may be imperfections, remember that facial beauty comes in all ages, shapes, and colors. Your face is an original—it is yours alone.

Although our differences are what makes each of us uniquely beautiful, one constant element that brings out our own distinctive beauty is healthy skin. Without it, the most elaborate makeup won't help you look your best. Beyond vanity, maintaining healthy skin is the body's primary line of defense against disease and infection.

The first step in creating beautiful, healthy skin is learning to read the messages your skin is sending you. Since your skin is a reflection of your general health, it follows that lack of sleep, hormonal swings, and other imbalances appear on your face first. The appearance of our skin can even point to more serious illness. In fact, for centuries, the Chinese have looked to the color of the skin surrounding the eyes as an indication of health problems. For example, a bluish cast can point to trouble with the kidneys. A green hue might be diagnosed as a liver imbalance.

Your face will also reveal your bad habits. Smoking and excessive sunbathing can prematurely age skin, leading to the early appearance of wrinkles. Alcohol, even in moderate amounts, can dehydrate the skin and interfere with your body's circulation. And if you're the type who thinks chocolate is one of the major food groups, your skin will rebel with bouts of excess oil and blemishes.

Stress can also have an adverse effect on the appearance of your skin. While we've all had days when worry and fatigue make us look less than glowing, when stress becomes the norm rather than the exception, our complexion suffers. Skin becomes dull and pasty, susceptible to breakouts.

To understand how to nurture a radiant complexion, it's important to know how the skin works. The skin is composed of three layers. The *epidermis* is the outermost layer of the skin. Often thought of as the protective layer, it is made up of dense protein cells known as keratin. These cells are shed every twenty-eight days, exposing the fresh, new skin that lies underneath. Below the epidermis is the *dermis*, a complex layer of blood vessels, hair follicles, and sebaceous (oil) glands that provide support to the skin. The dermis has a wonderful elastic quality to it thanks to a network of protein-based tissue called elastin and collagen. While these proteins can rejuvenate themselves, overexposure to the sun's rays will eventually destroy them, resulting in sagging skin and wrinkles. Providing nourishment to the dermis and epidermis, the bottom layer, or *hypodermis*, is made up of fatty tissue that retains body heat, protects the internal organs against trauma, and gives our skin its smooth appearance.

The skin is our largest organ—a living, breathing barrier against the environment; a complex system that releases toxins, maintains our body temperature, and prevents microorganisms from entering the body. It makes sense, then, to treat it kindly in an effort to maintain its health and integrity.

The High Price of a Pretty Face

It's a typical morning . . . you roll out of bed and stumble into the bathroom. After a few seconds of examining your reflection in the mirror, you reach for the cleansing lotion. Next comes the toner to close the pores. Finally, you smooth on your moisturizer—complete with an SPF-15 sunscreen to guard against the harsh elements you'll be facing. Your whole morning skin care routine takes just two minutes. Yet, in the two minutes it takes to clean and condition your skin, you might have exposed yourself to more than fifty synthetic chemicals.

At night, the routine begins again. You whisk away stale eye makeup with a convenient pad. Instead of your daytime moisturizer, you opt for a "nourishing" night cream or alpha hydroxy preparation. And just to be on the safe side, before sliding between the covers, you dab on a bit of specially formulated eye cream to ward off those dreaded crow's-feet.

Unfortunately, this type of daily cleansing and moisturizing exacts a high toll not just on your pocketbook but also on your appearance and your health. Conventional skin care products are packed with synthetic antibacterials, preservatives, thickeners, emulsifiers, colors, and fragrance that can irritate delicate skin and strip natural oils, making you look old before your time. These same ingredients may also be carcinogenic, disrupt your hormones, or cause an allergic reaction. Applied twice a day, day after day, these toxins are absorbed into your skin and make their way into your bloodstream.

Caustic Cleansers

As children, most of us were introduced to soap at a very young age. A little soap and water was the surest way to banish the grime accumulated during a busy day at play. But as we grew, we discovered that even the gentlest bar of soap was highly alkaline, leaving our skin taut and dry. So, we turned to the wonderful world of cleansers. Whether we chose a cream or lotion, cleansers promised to wash away dirt and impurities and leave our skin soft and clean.

While most commercial cleansing creams and lotions melt away dead skin cells and dislodge the dirt, they rely on alcohol and petroleum derivatives to get the job done. Alcohol is a solvent used widely in various forms, including ethyl, methyl, and cetyl alcohol. Since they dissolve fats (including the skin's natural oils), these alcohols can be very drying. To counteract the drying effects of alcohol, many manufacturers add mineral oil or petrolatum to leave the surface of skin feeling soft and pliant.

Other synthetic ingredients commonly found in cleansing creams and lotions include known or suspected carcinogens such as diethanolamine (DEA), triethanolamine (TEA), cocamide MEA, FD&C colors, and antibacterials. Hormone-disrupting parabens and formaldehyde-releasing preservatives such as DMDM hydantoin are common additions. Irritants and sensitizers such as PEG compounds, stearic acid, and synthetic perfumes are also frequently found in cleansing formulas.

Toxic Tighteners

While cleansers provide an alternative to harsh soaps, they can leave a residual film on our skin, making it look dull and even greasy. To whisk away the last traces of cleanser and dead skin cells, we reach for a skin-freshening toner or astringent.

Toners and astringents are often used interchangeably, yet they actually perform very different functions. Toners are ideally designed to refresh and "tone" the skin by closing the pores and balancing the skin's pH level. But a number of toners on the market today rely on plasticizers such as sorbitol and polyvinylpyrrolidone (PVP), a resin that can remain in the body for months after use, to produce that "tight" feeling.

Commercial astringents, on the other hand, often control the flow of oil with high concentrations of alcohol, which can disrupt the skin's natural pH balance. Because of the high alcohol content, astringents can dry even the oiliest complexion immediately after use. Yet, used daily, these products can actually increase oil production.

Along with alcohol, many over-the-counter astringents contain salicylic acid. While salicylic acid occurs naturally in wintergreen and sweet birch, the synthetic variety is prepared by heating phenol, sodium hydroxide, and carbon dioxide. Salicylic acid is toxic and contact with the skin should be avoided.

Another common ingredient in astringents is boric acid, an antiseptic with bactericidal and fungicidal properties. The American Medical Association (AMA) has warned of its possible toxicity and the Food and Drug Administration (FDA) issued a statement in 1992 saying that boric acid has not been show to be safe in over-the-counter products.[1]

Commercial toners and astringents can also contain talc, as well as synthetic colors, fragrance, and preservatives, making them potentially irritating. Safer and more soothing ways to tone your skin after cleansing include witch hazel and plain old water.

Lotions, Potions, and Miracle Creams

We all know that moisture is vital to keeping skin smooth, soft, and wrinkle-free. Maintaining the skin's moisture content not only makes us look better but also is important to the health of our skin. While we may forgo using a moisturizer when we're young, as we age, it becomes our best friend. We slather it on morning and night, hoping to stave off the effects of aging.

Our skin is constantly exposed to sun, wind, and arid indoor environments, conditions that can dehydrate the skin, aging it prematurely. Moisturizers are designed to prevent water loss by either coating the skin with an oily substance or coaxing water from the internal layers of the skin to the surface. A good moisturizer contains humectants, which boost the skin's ability to hold moisture. While nature provides a bounty of botanical humectants, including aloe vera, marshmallow, cucumber, calendula, and red sea algae, synthetic moisturizers are another story.

Relying on mainstream moisturizers and night creams may actually sabotage our skin's moisture content. Instead of natural oils and plant-based emollients, most brand-name moisturizers are packed with petrochemicals such as mineral oil and petrolatum. These refined crude oil products are blocking compounds that lie on the surface of skin, effectively preventing the skin's normal respiration. Since these compounds also clog our pores, they can prevent the release of toxins and waste. And, although all moisturizers make our skin feel smooth and soft immediately after we apply them, these synthetic compounds may actually pull moisture from the skin.

Virtually all popular moisturizers contain synthetic detergents, despite scientific evidence that these chemicals damage the skin and degrade the skin's natural protective function. Also damaging are the thickeners and plasticizers used to make the product rich and creamy.

Most of us are under the false impression that moisturizers not only keep our skin smooth and soft but also actually help heal the skin. However, recent studies have shown that many conventional moisturizers and emollients actually delay the healing of irritated and damaged skin by inhibiting the skin's natural ability to repair itself.

What about the new "nourishing" night creams? Heavier than traditional day creams, night creams are based on the same ingredients found in moisturizers but add wax esters such as beeswax or lanolin. Valued by cosmetics manufacturers for their emulsifying and humectant properties, DEA and TEA also find their way into a number of night creams. Although cosmetics companies promote these creams as suitable for nighttime use, the AMA's Committee on Cutaneous Health finds little difference between traditional moisturizers and night creams.[2]

The past few years have seen some major changes in moisturizing creams and lotions. Antioxidant herbs and vitamins, not to mention alpha hydroxy acids and sunscreens, have been added in an effort to keep the effects of aging at bay. Rushing to calm consumers' fears that aging invariably means tiny lines and wrinkles, manufacturers have developed high-tech serums, liposomes, silicon sheets, and nanospheres that promise to erase the years by reducing the appearance of these visible signs of aging.

Turning Back the Clock—Hope or Hype?

According to dermatologists and skin care manufacturers, hydroxy acids and topical vitamin creams can take years off your face. But in the ever-changing landscape of miracle creams, it's difficult to know which products actually live up to their claims.

Alpha hydroxy acids are weak acids that exfoliate the skin, essentially speeding up the process of sloughing off dead skin cells. This rapid smoothing of dry, rough skin diminishes visible lines and makes skin appear less wrinkled, which accounts for the huge success of these products in the marketplace.

AHAs, as they're commonly known, are nothing new. In fact, nature has provided this miracle since time began. Apples, grapes, black currants, and citrus fruits are rich in alpha hydroxy acids and have been used for centuries in natural skin care formulas. But the AHAs used in commercial antiaging creams have nothing to do with natural fruit acids. The most prominent ingredient used in over-the-counter alpha hydroxy preparations is glycolic acid. Although this chemical was originally derived from sugarcane, the glycolic acid in most AHA preparations is manufactured from chloracetic acid and salicylic acid, both synthetic creations of their natural counterparts.

The FDA has received more than a hundred complaints from consumers about AHAs burning and blistering the skin.[3] Even without these adverse reactions, overuse can irritate the skin and cause photosensitivity.

Perhaps the best-known and most effective AHA is tretinoin, commonly known as retin-A. Retin-A is a synthetic form of vitamin A and is available only by prescription. Studies have shown that retin-A can improve the appearance of surface wrinkles by increasing the turnover of cells, thickening the epidermis, and improving the texture of the skin. But don't be misled. The retinol or vitamin A listed on your over-the-counter antiwrinkle cream isn't the same as retin-A. Retinol, a derivative of vitamin A, is a completely different chemical. Although cosmetic manufacturers claim that retinol is the biggest cosmetic breakthrough in the fight against the signs of aging, the truth is that the research is inconclusive.

Despite the lack of hard evidence, topical vitamins have become the latest darling on the antiaging scene. Why are vitamins so critical to healthy skin? In our modern society, our skin is bombarded by the sun, pollution, the chlorine in drinking water, and even stress—all factors that contribute to the production of free radicals. Although free radicals are naturally occurring by-products of a variety of physical reactions, when the body is overwhelmed by these substances, they oxidize and become toxic, accelerating the aging process. Free radicals attack healthy skin cells, damaging the DNA and RNA in the cell nuclei. They also chew up collagen, the genetic glue that holds the skin together and keeps it firm and supple. The most effective way to fight this oxidative damage is with antioxidant vitamins. Antioxidants block the oxidation process, destroying free radicals before they can do any harm.

Traditionally, antioxidants have been taken orally, either in food or in supplements. But recently, they've been showing up in skin care products, particularly vitamins A, C, and E. The theory behind including antioxidant vitamins in skin care treatments is simple: although vitamins when taken orally are particularly good at protecting the body from free radical damage, as we age, these vitamins have a harder time reaching the skin. "Even if you have an adequate supply of antioxidants in your blood, that doesn't mean your skin is getting its fair share," notes Lorraine Meisner, Ph.D., a geneticist at the University of Wisconsin. "As we get older, the tiny vessels in the skin become compromised and aren't able to feed the skin."[4] Malnourished and sun-damaged skin is a prime target for free radicals. Researchers believe that applying antioxidant agents directly to the skin will make them more available where they are needed most.

Although more research is needed, the studies that have been conducted concerning the effectiveness of vitamins A, C, and E look promising. "The antioxidant properties of these three vitamins may work when applied topically to fight signs of photoaging," says Karen Keller, M.D., in a study published by the American Academy of Dermatology. "Many patients note improvement in skin texture, wrinkles, and age spots while using these products."[5]

How well the new over-the-counter vitamin creams work to restore the skin's ability to repair itself depends on their ability to penetrate the skin. While vitamin E seems to penetrate the skin fairly easily, vitamin C must first be encapsulated in liposomes, minuscule fat sacs that supposedly slide through the skin's surface like a hot knife through butter.

Concentration is also an issue. Experts are hotly debating how much of a vitamin is needed to begin cellular repair, especially vitamin C. While some believe a 10 percent vitamin C concentration has the ability to stimulate collagen, others feel that lower concentrations (1 to 3 percent) can effectively reduce the effects of photoaging.

Another problem is stability. According to Steven Lamm, M.D., clinical assistant professor of medicine at New York University's School of Medicine, it's a delicate balance: "A low pH or acidity level helps vitamin C remain stable. On the other hand, if the pH is too low, it can burn the skin."[6] The problem with choosing a vitamin cream off the shelf is that it may not state the pH level. If you have sensitive skin, you may want to patch-test the product before use.

Another way to give your skin the benefit of antioxidants is with botanicals. Long before synthetic vitamins made their appearance at cosmetics counters, women indigenous to tropical rain forests used plants and herbs to tame the signs of aging. Today, Japanese scientists have confirmed that several herbs are potent antioxidants, including horse chestnut, witch hazel, rosemary, and sage. Green tea extract, grape seed oil, and chamomile are also valued by natural skin care manufacturers for their antioxidant properties. Incorporated into skin creams, these natural antioxidants may be more readily absorbed than their synthetic counterparts.

The newest antioxidant to show up in natural antiaging cosmetics is pyc-nogenol, a bioflavonoid compound derived from the French maritime pine. Advocates say pycnogenol improves skin elasticity and strengthens capillaries, although there is little research to back up these claims.

While hard scientific research hasn't caught up with the anecdotal evidence of botanical antioxidants, Dr. Meisner says, "If nothing else, these ingredients can help maintain the potency of the vitamins in a product."

Sun Sense

Since AHAs and topical vitamins can reduce the appearance of wrinkles only temporarily, it's important to do whatever we can to prevent them in the first place. Wrinkles and other signs of aging aren't inevitable—prematurely aged skin is a direct result of too much sun. And overexposure significantly raises the risk of developing skin cancer. Yet, we need a certain amount of exposure to ensure the production of vitamin D and to maintain mental and emotional health. What to do? *Wear sunscreen.* It's a mantra shared by dermatologists and skin care specialists across the country. This advice has blossomed into a booming sideline for cosmetics manufacturers, which include sunscreens in everything from moisturizers to foundations to lipstick.

Sun-protection products are broken down into two basic categories—physical and chemical. Physical blocks, more commonly known as sunblocks, work as a barrier against sun damage. The best-known sunblock is zinc oxide, a naturally occurring mineral that has been found to be more effective than some chemical ingredients at blocking out the sun's harmful rays.[7] Although some sunblocks include chemical filters, red petroleum, and talc, products without these synthetic ingredients are generally safe and nonirritating.

Chemical blocks, better known as sunscreens, work by absorbing most of the sun's ultraviolet rays before they reach the skin. For years, para-aminobenzoic acid, or PABA, was the most effective chemical for screening out harmful ultraviolet rays. But PABA, one of the B vitamins, proved too harsh for many users, and although some brands still include PABA in their products, a number of manufacturers are now offering "PABA-free" sunscreens to minimize adverse reactions.

While all chemical sunscreens filter out the painful burning rays called ultraviolet B (UVB), some of the newer products employ benzophonones and cinnamates to guard against ultraviolet A (UVA) rays, which penetrate the epidermal layer, attacking the deeper levels of the skin. Labeled "broad-spectrum" sunscreens, these products are supposed to provide the maximum screening protection from both UVA and UVB rays.

Although most dermatologists recommend using a product with a rating of SPF-15, when it comes to sunscreens, most of us are confused by the term. SPF, or sun protection factor, simply refers to the amount of time you can safely stay out in the sun. For example, "If, without any sunscreen, you would ordinarily burn after ten minutes of exposure to the sun, a sunscreen with an SPF value of 6 would protect you six times longer," explains David M. Stoll, M.D., author of *A Woman's Skin* and a fellow of the American Academy of Dermatology.[8]

Are these chemical sunscreens really a cure-all in the prevention of pho-todamaged skin? When it comes to preventing certain skin cancers, not all scientists agree. "Sunscreens have—at least in theory—the potential to inflict damage," says Dr. John Knowland of the University of Oxford, whose research indicates that sunscreens containing PABA and its derivatives, such as padimate-O, can damage DNA. He adds, "Since sunscreens are so widely used, it's important to know as much as possible about them."[9] Yet, surprisingly few studies on the safety of sunscreens have been published. And what has been published is virtually ignored by both the media and the medical community. One study conducted by the University of Queensland found that significant amounts of oxybenzone, a common sunscreen ingredient, appear to penetrate the epidermal barrier.[10]

Much of the controversy over the safety of chemical sunscreens stems from the parallel rise in sunscreen use and skin cancer. In fact, University of California, San Diego, epidemiologists Cedric and Frank Garland believe that the increased use of chemical sunscreens since the mid-1970s is the primary cause of the current skin cancer epidemic. The Garlands suggest that sunscreen use, and the prolonged sunbathing it allows, may lead to melanoma, the deadliest form of skin cancer.[11]

Because of consumer confusion over SPFs, many people buy a sunscreen with an SPF rating of 30 or above; yet, according to a recent study by the European Institute of Oncology, most sun worshipers don't use enough sunscreen to reach the levels of sun protection indicated on the label. Although the Skin Cancer Foundation recommends using at least one full ounce, or the equivalent of a shot glass, most consumers use only 25 to 30 percent of the recommended amount. Consequently, say the researchers, an SPF-50 sunscreen applied at this reduced thickness yields a practical SPF of about 2. They go on to state that the current SPF system is misleading, since it doesn't reflect actual usage, and call for a change in how SPFs are measured.[12] Although the FDA is working to ban the labeling of sunscreens with a rating of SPF-30 and higher, the Cosmetic, Toiletry, and Fragrance Association and several sun care manufacturers have cried foul and have succeeded in pushing back the final ruling on this critical issue.[13]

In February 1998, epidemiologist Marianne Berwick of the Memorial Sloan-Kettering Cancer Center in New York presented an evaluation of several studies of sunscreen use and cancer at an annual meeting of the American Association for the Advancement of Sciences and concluded that there is no scientific evidence that the use of sunscreen actually prevents skin cancer.[14] Dr. Gordon Ainsleigh agrees, estimating that thirty thousand cancer deaths in the United States could be prevented each year if people would adopt a regimen of regular, but moderate, sun exposure instead of relying on the heavy use of sunscreens. In an article published in *Preventative Medicine*, Dr. Ainsleigh went so far as to propose that the use of sunscreen causes more cancer deaths than it prevents.[15]

Although the jury is still out on this critical issue, there are some sensible measures you can take to minimize the risks of photodamaged skin and skin cancer. First, limit your exposure to twenty to thirty minutes a day, avoiding the hours between 11:00 A.M. and 2:00 P.M. If you know you're going to be exposed for longer periods, opt for a mineral-based sunblock product and wear a wide-brimmed hat to shade the delicate facial skin.

Getting to Know Your Skin

In skin care circles, everything depends on your skin type. Knowing what type of skin you have helps you choose products that will actually nourish and support your individual complexion. Too often, women rely on a friend's recommendation or industry advertising when choosing cleansing and moisturizing products, without taking into account the individuality of their own skin.

If you're not sure what type of skin you have, try this: Wash your face before bedtime to remove any traces of dirt, oil, and makeup. Resist the urge to apply moisturizer, night cream, or any other product you normally use. Before washing your face the next morning, press a piece of tissue paper or brown wrapping paper on your face, especially your chin, nose, and forehead (the T-zone). If the paper doesn't show any oily residue, you have dry skin. Normal skin will leave a small amount of oil, and oily skin will leave a definite stain.

While this little experiment will give you a good idea of what type of skin you have, Table 4.1 will acquaint you with the nuances of each type.

Table 4.1 ❧ Getting to Know Your Face

Dry Skin:	Dry skin is delicate and thin, with a fine texture and no visible pores. Tight and dry, especially after washing, dry skin can become flaky and more susceptible to wrinkles. Fair complexions often tend to be dry.
Normal Skin:	Normal skin contains just the right balance of oil. Smooth and supple, normal skin is not prone to blemishes. If you have normal skin, count your blessings. The rest of us would kill for your complexion!
Oily Skin:	Oily skin tends to be shiny and has larger pores, thanks to overactive oil glands. Without proper maintenance, this abundance of oil can result in eruptions. The good news is that oily skin is more resistant to sun damage, harsh treatment, and wrinkles than is dry skin.
Combination Skin:	Combination skin is just that—a combination of skin types. Your forehead, nose, and chin are oily, while your cheeks are tight and dry. Unless your T-zone is excessively oily, most dermatologists recommend following a skin care routine designed for normal complexions.

Skin Smarts: Pampering Your Face Naturally

Once you've determined what type of skin you have, the next step is to create a customized daily skin care routine that's right for your skin. But no matter what your skin type, the basics for every skin care routine revolve around three elements: cleansing, toning, and moisturizing.

Cleansing is critical to glowing skin. It removes dirt, dead skin cells, makeup, and excess oil. But, as we've seen, not all cleansers are designed to protect delicate facial skin. Soaps can be harsh, and synthetic cleansers can actually dry skin. But natural cleansers are formulated to dissolve and wash away impurities without disrupting the skin's natural acid mantle.

Cleansers come in the form of creams, milks, gels, or foaming compounds. Whichever type you use, gently massage a small amount into your face, using small circular motions. After a minute or so, rinse well with tepid water or wipe away the excess with damp cotton. Never use a washcloth on your face since the rough fabric can damage the delicate connective facial tissue.

To ensure that all traces of cleanser and dirt are removed, follow your cleanser with a good toner. Toners rebalance the skin's pH and refine the pores. Ideally, toners should be splashed, dabbed, or misted onto the face. Aloe vera juice, witch hazel, and weak herbal vinegar are all good natural toners.

Finally, use a moisturizer designed to protect the skin without clogging the pores. Since moisturizers work more effectively when the skin is slightly damp, applying your moisturizer immediately after cleansing and toning will help it penetrate the skin.

Simply dab a bit of moisturizer on your cheeks, chin, nose, and forehead, and gently massage it into your skin. Wait a few minutes for the moisturizer to be absorbed before applying makeup. Following this routine morning and night helps to prevent impurities from becoming lodged in your pores, where they can lead to dull skin, blemishes, and premature wrinkles.

Special Treatments

A regular skin care routine will go a long way toward maintaining healthy, beautiful skin, but periodically our skin needs a bit of extra care. Exfoliating, steaming, and using facial masks can all benefit the skin, especially as we age. Since the skin begins to deteriorate by the time a woman reaches her thirtieth birthday, this extra care can help to fend off the signs of aging. These treatments can be incorporated into your skin care routine on a weekly or monthly basis.

Exfoliating

Mechanical exfoliation removes accumulated dead skin cells, leaving you with a softer, smoother complexion. Don't confuse mechanical exfoliation with the exfoliation that occurs when you use AHAs. Mechanical exfoliators are creams or lotions containing cleansing grains—fine, sandlike particles that have a mild abrasive action on the skin. Commonly called facial scrubs, these products are designed to loosen debris from the surface of the skin and stimulate circulation.

Unfortunately, most commercial scrubs contain harsh alcohols and detergents, DEA, TEA, or sodium lauryl sulfate, not to mention an array of synthetic colors, scents, and preservatives. Instead of scrubbing your face with chemicals, try cornmeal. Cornmeal is an excellent natural exfoliant that removes dead skin cells and helps to unclog pores. Simply moisten your skin and gently massage a bit of cornmeal into your face, using a circular motion. Rinse thoroughly with tepid water for glowing skin.

Steaming

Steaming is another skin care basic. A facial steam won't remove dirt and grime, but it will soften the surface of the skin enough to help unclog pores. Steaming your face will also increase circulation and humidify the skin.

To give yourself a facial steam, bring a large pot of water to a boil. Cover your head with a bath towel to form a tent, and hold your face ten to twelve inches from the top of the pot. Allow the steam to work for ten minutes. For a special aromatherapeutic treat or to address a specific condition such as acne, add a handful of fragrant herbs to the boiling water. Skin-friendly antiseptic herbs suitable for steaming include lavender, rose petals, geranium, and rosemary. Chamomile and calendula are also useful for soothing an irritated complexion.

While steaming is good for all skin types, if you have broken capillaries, it's a good idea to avoid this treatment.

Facial Masks

Masks have been used for centuries to moisturize, stimulate, and cleanse the skin. Masks come in a variety of formulas, depending on the results desired: moisturizing, tightening, cleansing, stimulating, or nourishing.

The two basic types of masks are clay-based and cream masks. Clay-based masks are the most astringent of all mask formulations. This type of mask is valued for its ability to absorb oil and pull dirt and toxins from the skin. Clay masks also stimulate the circulation and tighten the pores.

To use a clay mask, simply mix the clay with enough water or apple cider vinegar to form a paste, and apply the mixture to the skin in an even layer. Allow the mask to remain in place for fifteen to thirty minutes until it is almost dry, before thoroughly rinsing with tepid water. Unlike mainstream clay masks, which often include propylene glycol, alcohol, diazolidinyl urea, and artificial colors, the natural masks available in health food stores are based on kaolin or bentonite clay.

Cream masks, on the other hand, are designed to moisturize and nourish the skin. They are nondrying and are good for dry, mature, or sensitive skin. Although commercial cream masks often contain many of the same synthetic ingredients found in conventional moisturizers and night creams, natural cream masks are usually based on herbs containing soothing, emollient properties.

One simple moisturizing mask you can try at home is plain yogurt. Apply an even layer of room-temperature yogurt to the face, and rinse well after ten to fifteen minutes. For added moisture, mix a tablespoon of aloe vera into the yogurt. To treat a specific problem, you can also add one of the herbs or essential oils described in Table 4.2.

Troubleshooting Troubled Skin

No matter how diligent we are, age, stress, and pollutants can wreak havoc with our complexion. Here are a few of the more common problems to which we are all subject:

Acne

Contrary to popular belief, pimples and blackheads are not reserved for teenagers. Acne can crop up later in life as a response to fluctuating estrogen levels, particularly during pregnancy and menopause. Acne can also be a sign of poor elimination or a buildup of toxins.

Acne occurs when excess oil production combines with dead skin cells to clog pores. Clogged pores are a breeding ground for bacteria and can result in red inflamed pimples, pus-filled whiteheads, or unsightly blackheads.

Cosmetics counters are littered with acne treatments, most containing strong chemicals such as salicylic acid or benzoyl peroxide. Available in creams or medicated pads, these products can actually exacerbate the problem by irritating the skin. Instead of using harsh chemicals to banish acne, try a bit of tea tree oil. Not only is the essential oil less irritating, but also a study conducted by King's College in London found tea tree oil to be an effective antimicrobial treatment for acne.[16]

The most important step in managing acne is maintaining scrupulously clean skin. Antibacterial, anti-inflammatory herbs can also be useful in treating the occasional blemish. Applying a dab of lavender, geranium, or chamomile essential oil can reduce swelling and redness and aid in healing. Rubbing the affected area with the cut side of a clove of raw garlic can also stop a blemish from blossoming into a full-blown crisis. Astringent herbs such as bergamot, juniper, lemongrass, rose, and sandalwood may also be helpful in controlling oil production. For more severe cases, the antibiotic properties in goldenseal and echinacea can be helpful when applied topically.

While these herbs may be incorporated into facial creams, masks, and steam treatments, you can also dilute their essential oils in a carrier oil for spot treatment.

Although you've probably been told a hundred times, it bears repeating: never squeeze a pimple. Squeezing and picking at pimples and blackheads will irritate them and increase inflammation. In fact, the residue that remains after "popping" a pimple will only cause more eruptions.

Freckles and Age Spots

For years, mothers have tried to convince their daughters that freckles give a face personality. Some of us agreed, but many women will try anything and everything to rid their skin of freckles.

Freckles are caused by the skin's effort to tan in spots where there is an uneven distribution of melanin. Age or liver spots, on the other hand, are a delayed reaction to sun exposure and usually don't appear until our forties or fifties.

The use of vanishing or bleaching creams is a popular way to try to reverse these sun-induced imperfections. Before 1973, many vanishing creams contained ammoniated mercury, a poisonous substance that has since been banned by the FDA.[17] Today, manufacturers have replaced the lethal mercury compound with hydroquinone. Although legal in the eyes of the FDA, hydroquinone is made from crystalline phenol and is toxic. A suspected carcinogen, hydroquinone may also cause allergic reactions.[18] Long-term use can result in blotches, yellowish brown bumps, and eventually scarring.

For a safer method of fading freckles and age spots, apply undiluted lemon juice. Not only does lemon juice have bleaching properties, but it also acts as a mild exfoliant. If you have sensitive skin, dilute the lemon juice in an equal amount of water before application.

Regardless of the method, the bleaching of skin discoloration is a long-term proposition. It can take months before you notice any lightening, and once the treatment is stopped, the spots will reappear.

Broken Capillaries

Tiny red lines around the nose and cheeks, commonly called thread veins, can plague any type of skin, but people with thin, delicate, or mature skin are more prone to this condition. If you suffer from broken capillaries, avoid extreme water temperatures when you wash your face since this can bring the blood to the surface of the skin, making the problem worse. It's also a good idea to avoid facial scrubs and astringent masks, which increase circulation. And never scrub your face with a rough washcloth or loofah. Instead, opt for the gentlest skin care products you can find, preferably products containing yogurt, papaya, or aloe vera.

You can also strengthen capillaries with herbs. Calendula, ginkgo biloba, lavender, rose, and neroli can strengthen capillaries while soothing irritated skin and reducing inflammation. A chamomile infusion used daily as a compress can also reduce thread veins.

Table 4.2 lists numerous useful home remedies for a variety of skin problems.

Homemade Skin Care

Keeping your skin clean, soft, and healthy is an individual pursuit. Fortunately, making your own skin care products gives you the freedom to customize products for your own skin type and problems—a benefit you'll never get from mass-marketed products.

Table 4.2 ❧ Herbal Remedies for Skin

Customized skin preparations can cost a fortune. By learning which herbs and essential oils benefit your particular skin type, you can search out off-the-shelf products that contain these ingredients . . . or create your own custom blend for a truly nontoxic treat.

If You Have . . .	Useful Herbs	Comments and Cautions
acne	burdock, calendula, garlic, lavender, lemon, nasturtium, rosemary, sage, Saint-John's-wort, tea tree, thyme	
age spots	horseradish, lemon	Horseradish may irritate, even burn, sensitive skin.
blotchy skin	aloe vera, horse chestnut, Saint-John's-wort	
chapped skin	cucumber, geranium, marshmallow, rose, slippery elm	
dark circles	hops, stinging nettle, witch hazel	
dermatitis	aloe vera, benzoin, chamomile, lavender, melissa, patchouli, rose, ylang-ylang	
dry skin	cucumber, rose, slippery elm	
eczema	chamomile, geranium, marshmallow, melissa, rosemary	
fragile capillaries	chamomile, juniper, neroli, rose, witch hazel	
irritated skin	aloe vera, chamomile, calendula	
itchy skin	aloe vera, chamomile	
oily skin	burdock, eyebright, honeysuckle, sage, witch hazel, yarrow	
pimples	echinacea, garlic, lavender, parsley, peppermint, tea tree	

If You Have . . .	Useful Herbs	Comments and Cautions
puffy eyes	chamomile	
rash	aloe vera, chamomile	If the rash persists, seek medical attention.
sensitive skin	chamomile, jasmine, neroli, rose, Saint-John's-wort, witch hazel	
sunburn	aloe vera, benzoin, bilberry, chamomile, echinacea, horse chestnut	Apple cider vinegar will also soothe a painful sunburn.
wrinkles	chamomile, cypress, frankincense, ginseng, gotu kola, horsetail, neroli, rose, sandalwood	

Cleansers

Removing dirt and impurities on a daily basis is crucial to the health of your skin. Since many of the following cleansers include fresh fruits, vegetables, and dairy products, refrigeration is essential.

Dry Skin Cleanser   YIELD: 3 ounces
The aloe vera, glycerin, and jojoba moisturize dry skin.

   ¼ cup aloe vera gel
   1 teaspoon jojoba oil
   1 teaspoon glycerin
   ½ teaspoon grapefruit seed extract
   8 drops sandalwood essential oil
   4 drops rosemary essential oil
   1 capsule vitamin E

Mix the ingredients with a wire whisk until blended. To use, apply with a cotton ball. Rinse well with warm water. Since this mixture tends to separate, shake well before each use.

Oily Skin Cleanser

YIELD: 3 ounces

The astringent properties in this cleanser help control excess oil. This cleanser needs no refrigeration.

- ¼ cup witch hazel
- 1 teaspoon apple cider vinegar
- 1 teaspoon glycerin
- ½ teaspoon grapefruit seed extract
- 6 drops lemon essential oil
- 4 drops sage essential oil
- 1 capsule vitamin E

Mix the ingredients with a wire whisk until blended. To use, apply with a cotton ball. Rinse well with warm water.

Blemish Busting Cleanser

YIELD: 3 ounces

Lavender's antiseptic and anti-inflammatory properties help speed the healing of problem skin.

- ¼ cup witch hazel
- 1 teaspoon glycerin
- ½ teaspoon grapefruit seed extract
- 8 drops lavender essential oil
- 4 drops tea tree essential oil
- 1 capsule vitamin E

Mix the ingredients with a wire whisk until blended. To use, apply with a cotton ball. Rinse well with warm water.

Easy Oatmeal Cleanser

YIELD: 1 cup

The easiest of all cleansers. Oatmeal not only cleans away surface dirt but also softens the skin.

- 1 cup rolled oats

Place the oats in a blender and process until fine. Keep in a jar or bowl next to your sink. To use, scoop a small amount of the oatmeal into your hand and gently massage into your wet skin. Rinse with warm water.

Strawberry Fields Cleanser   YIELD: 5 ounces

This cleanser has a mild astringent action. Slippery elm is included to balance the styptic properties of the strawberries and witch hazel.

6 whole strawberries
6 strawberry leaves
3 tablespoons witch hazel
2 tablespoons almond oil
½ teaspoon slippery elm

Place the ingredients in a blender or food processor and blend until smooth. Transfer the mixture to a clean jar. To use, gently massage a small amount into your skin, using a circular motion. Rinse well with warm water.

Citrus Cleansing Milk   YIELD: 3 ounces

A cleanser and toner in one. This moisturizing formula is good for dry skin.

½ cup plain yogurt
1½ teaspoons lemon juice
1 tablespoon jojoba oil
5 drops lemon essential oil

Using a blender or food processor, blend the yogurt and lemon juice. While the machine is running, slowly add the jojoba oil, and mix until smooth. Transfer the mixture to a clean jar and stir in the lemon essential oil. To use, gently massage a small amount into your skin, using a circular motion. Rinse well with warm water.

Facial Scrubs

While cleansers remove surface dirt, scrubs are good for those times when deeper cleaning is called for. Since scrubs are, by nature, more abrasive than cleansers, don't use them more than once a week.

Corn Nut Facial Scrub   YIELD: 1 cup

This is a basic, all-purpose scrub.

½ cup cornmeal
½ cup almond meal
1 teaspoon chamomile flowers

Mix the ingredients together. Keep in a jar or bowl next to your sink. To use, scoop a small amount into your hand and gently massage into wet skin. Rinse with warm water.

Rose Petal Scrub   YIELD: 5 ounces
Rose has a soothing and moisturizing effect on the skin.

- 2 tablespoons oatmeal
- 2 tablespoons ground almonds
- 2 tablespoons rose petals
- 4 drops rose essential oil

Mix the oatmeal, almonds, and rose petals in a small bowl. Add the essential oil, stirring to disperse. To use, gently massage into skin, using a circular motion. Rinse well with warm water.

Simple Sugar Scrub   YIELD: 4 ounces
One of the best alpha hydroxy acids, glycolic acid, is derived from sugarcane. This scrub combines the best of mechanical and chemical exfoliants and leaves your skin incredibly soft and smooth.

- ¼ cup white cane sugar
- ¼ cup avocado oil
- ½ teaspoon vitamin C crystals
- 2 drops rose essential oil

Combine the ingredients in a small bowl. Massage a small amount into your face, using circular motions. After a few minutes, rinse well with warm water. Store any leftover scrub in the refrigerator.

Astringents, Toners, and Skin Fresheners

Toners and skin fresheners are best for normal to dry skin. Astringents, on the other hand, are very acidic and may contain alcohol. They are best suited to oily skin.

Rose Water   YIELD: 17 ounces
Rose water was a valued skin toner and softener during Victorian times. If you have roses in the garden, consider making it yourself since commercial brands can be expensive.

2 cups distilled water
¼ cup vodka
½ cup rose petals
15 drops rose essential oil

Mix the water, vodka, and rose petals in a large bowl. Pour into a clean glass bottle and set out in the sun for a day or two. Strain to remove petals. Add the rose essential oil and shake well to mix. This mixture can either be used as is to soothe sensitive skin or added to other formulas.

Herbal Toner for Dry Skin
YIELD: 4 ounces

This nondrying toner is ideal for dry, flaky skin.

¼ cup aloe vera juice
¼ cup rose water
6 drops rose geranium essential oil
4 drops sandalwood essential oil
1 drop chamomile essential oil
1 drop jasmine essential oil

Pour the ingredients into a clean glass bottle and shake to blend. Apply with a clean cotton ball.

Lemon Splash
YIELD: 5 ounces

A refreshing astringent with a delicate citrus scent.

½ cup witch hazel
4 teaspoons orange flower water
10 drops lemon essential oil

Pour the witch hazel and orange flower water into a clean glass bottle. Add the lemon essential oil, cap and shake to blend. Apply with a clean cotton ball.

Healing Toner for Sensitive Skin
YIELD: 5 ounces

For people blessed with an oily and sensitive complexion, this astringent toner removes excess oil while being gentle to the skin.

¼ cup rose water
2 tablespoons witch hazel
4 drops rose essential oil
2 drops yarrow essential oil

Mix the ingredients together in a clean glass bottle. Shake well to blend. Apply with a cotton ball.

Chamomile Astringent for Oily Skin   YIELD: 5 ounces
Tea tree oil is a wonderful antiseptic for problem skin.

> 1 cup witch hazel
> ½ teaspoon tea tree essential oil
> ½ cup chamomile tea

Pour the ingredients into a clean glass bottle. Shake to blend. Apply with a cotton ball.

Moisturizers

Moisturizers are surprisingly easy to make at home. Emollient herbs can be incorporated into homemade moisturizers to boost their effectiveness. Borage, marshmallow, rose petals, and slippery elm will all soften and soothe the skin. Since moisturizers can become rancid quickly, prepare them in small batches and be sure to keep them refrigerated. Use any of the moisturizers listed here as you would a commercial preparation.

Soothing Herbal Moisturizer   YIELD: 4½ ounces
This dry-skin moisturizer is packed with emollient-rich herbs.

> ½ cup aloe vera gel
> 1 tablespoon dried lavender flowers
> 1 tablespoon dried calendula flowers
> ½ teaspoon slippery elm
> 5 drops lavender essential oil

Combine the aloe vera gel, lavender flowers, calendula flowers, and slippery elm in a small pan. Heat gently over a low flame, stirring constantly. Remove from the heat and strain into a small bowl. Add the essential oil and mix thoroughly. Pour the finished moisturizer into a small jar and cap tightly.

Skin-Specific Herbal Moisturizer   YIELD: 3 ounces

This moisturizer can be formulated for different skin types. For dry skin, use an infusion of rose or geranium. For oily skin, try bergamot or juniper. Normal and problem skin will benefit from an infusion of lavender.

   2 ounces herbal infusion
   ½ ounce beeswax, grated
   1 tablespoon avocado oil
   2 teaspoons wheat germ oil
   5 drops essential oil (see recipe introduction)

Prepare the herbal infusion of your choice and set aside. Melt the beeswax in the top of a double boiler. Slowly add the avocado oil and wheat germ oil, beating constantly with a wooden spoon until incorporated. Remove the mixture from the heat and slowly add the herbal infusion, stirring constantly. Cool slightly and add the essential oil, mixing well. Immediately pour into a clean jar. Cool and cap tightly.

Nourishing Night Lotion   YIELD: 7 ounces

This vitamin-rich lotion softens the skin while it nourishes.

   1 tablespoon vitamin E oil
   1 tablespoon olive oil
   1 tablespoon avocado oil
   1 teaspoon wheat germ oil
   1 teaspoon liquid lecithin
   1 tablespoon beeswax, grated
   ½ cup purified water
   ½ teaspoon liquid vitamin C
   5 drops rose essential oil

Mix the avocado oil, wheat germ oil, lecithin, and beeswax in the top of a double boiler and heat gently until the beeswax has melted. Meanwhile, heat the water just to the boiling point. Remove the oil mixture from the heat and slowly add it to the water, stirring vigorously, or use a blender to mix. Add the vitamin C and essential oil. Stir to blend before pouring into a clean jar. Allow the mixture to cool, and cap with a tight-fitting lid.

Rose Day Cream
YIELD: 4 ounces

This rich yet light moisturizer not only soothes and softens the skin but also allows makeup to glide on.

¼ cup almond oil
1 tablespoon beeswax, grated
¼ cup rose water
5 drops rose essential oil

Combine the oil and beeswax in the top of a double boiler and heat until the beeswax has melted. Remove from the heat and add the rose water and essential oil, stirring constantly. Pour into a clean jar and allow to cool, stirring several times to prevent the mixture from separating. Cap with a tight-fitting lid.

Facial Masks

Facial masks are a wonderful way to perk up your complexion and give it a healthy glow. Since freshness is essential when using food-based masks, these masks should be made just before using.

Cleansing Meringue Mask
YIELD: 1 application

This healing mask clears away impurities and tightens pores. Great for oily skin!

2 egg whites
1 vitamin E capsule

Combine the egg whites and vitamin E in a large bowl and whip until stiff peaks form. Spread the mixture evenly onto the face and allow the mask to dry. Rinse thoroughly with tepid water.

Garden of Eden Mask
YIELD: 1 application

This nourishing mask is good for dry or sensitive skin.

1 ripe banana or avocado
1 vitamin E capsule

Mash the banana or avocado into a smooth paste. Drizzle the vitamin E over the fruit and blend well. Smooth evenly over face and neck. After 30 minutes, rinse well with tepid water until all traces of the mask have been removed.

Oatmeal and Honey Mask
YIELD: 1 application

Stimulates, tightens, and tones the complexion. A good choice for combination skin.

½ cup oatmeal
2 tablespoons honey

Blend the ingredients together and spread evenly over the face. Let the mask work for at least 30 minutes before rinsing well with tepid water.

Astringent Blemish Mask
YIELD: 1 application

This stimulating mask actually removes excess oil while pulling impurities from the skin, making it a good choice for problem skin. Note: This mask may be too astringent for sensitive skin.

2 tablespoons bentonite clay
2 tablespoons apple cider vinegar
7 drops lavender essential oil

Combine the ingredients in a glass bowl, stirring with a wooden spoon until a smooth paste has formed. Immediately spread a thin, even layer over your face and relax for 15 to 30 minutes. You will feel a tight, tingling sensation as the mask dries. Rinse thoroughly with tepid water. Your face may be slightly red immediately after using this mask.

Alpha Hydroxy Enzyme Mask
YIELD: 1 application

This is an excellent exfoliating mask.

½ ripe papaya
4 strawberries
1 tablespoon brewer's yeast

Cube the papaya and strawberries and process in a blender until smooth. Pour into a small bowl and mix in the brewer's yeast. Apply evenly to the face and neck. Allow the mask to remain on the face for 10 minutes before rinsing thoroughly with tepid water.

Quick Exfoliating Mask
YIELD: 1 application

Try this 5-minute mask to stimulate a sallow complexion and get rid of dead skin cells.

¼ cup baking soda
Purified water

Mix the baking soda with enough water to form a paste. Apply evenly to the face. After 5 minutes, rinse well with tepid water.

Facial Mists

Facial mists are a wonderfully refreshing way to keep your skin hydrated. They have the added benefit of setting makeup after application. Use these mists frequently if you have dry skin or spend a lot of time in artificially heated environments or traveling on airplanes.

Herbal Mist   YIELD: 4 ounces

While a spray bottle filled with purified water can be used to hydrate the skin, the addition of beneficial essential oils aids certain skin conditions and will give you an aromatherapeutic lift.

   ½ cup purified water
   10 drops essential oil

Combine the water and essential oil in a small spray bottle. Shake well to mix. To apply, spray a fine mist onto the face.
    Which essential oil should you include in your facial mist? Each of the following essential oils will target a specific skin condition:

Jasmine	Soothes and moisturizes dry skin.
Lavender	Antibacterial and anti-inflammatory. Good for acne.
Lemon	Stimulates aging skin.
Rose	Moisturizing. Promotes the formation of new cells. Good for sensitive or dry skin.

Special Treatments

Although nothing can take the place of proper skin care, occasionally we need a more intensive treatment. The treatments in this final section target specific problems.

Wrinkle Treatment
YIELD: 4 ounces

This is a good treatment following the use of alpha hydroxy acids. The healing properties of comfrey and witch hazel soothe aging skin, while the patchouli essential oil encourages the regeneration of skin cells.

¼ cup comfrey infusion
¼ cup witch hazel
10 drops patchouli essential oil

Combine the ingredients and store in a clean bottle. To use, apply to affected areas with a clean cotton ball.

Eye Cream
YIELD: 2 ounces

Used on a regular basis, this heavy cream will help chase away those dreaded crow's-feet.

1 teaspoon apricot kernel oil
1 teaspoon beeswax, grated
½ teaspoon aloe vera gel
3 drops grapefruit seed essential oil
1 vitamin E capsule

Combine the oil and beeswax in the top of a double boiler. Heat until the wax has melted and remove from the heat. Using a wooden spoon, beat in the aloe vera gel. Allow to cool slightly and add the essential oil and vitamin E, stirring well. Pour into a small jar. Cool and cap tightly.

Age Spot Vanishing Treatment
YIELD: 1 ounce

This treatment must be used daily for several months before any improvement is seen. Note: This is a fairly strong treatment. If burning or irritation occurs, discontinue use.

1 teaspoon horseradish, grated
1 teaspoon aloe vera gel
½ teaspoon fresh lemon juice
½ teaspoon white vinegar
3 drops lemon essential oil

Combine the ingredients, mixing well. Be careful not to touch the eyes after handling the grated horseradish, as it can result in severe burning. Set the mixture aside for 30 minutes before straining and pouring into a clean jar with a tight-fitting lid. To use, dab a bit of the solution on the affected area, using a clean cotton ball.

Instant Blemish Buster   YIELD: 2 ounces
This spot treatment will dry blemishes while reducing pain and inflammation.

> ¼ cup purified water
> 1 teaspoon Epsom salts
> 6 drops lavender essential oil
> 3 drops tea tree oil

Bring the water to a boil. Add the Epsom salts and stir to dissolve. Remove from heat and add the essential oils. To use, dip a clean cloth in the hot solution and apply to the affected area. When the cloth begins to cool, repeat the procedure. Do this several times.

Intensive Acne Treatment   YIELD: 1 ounce
This healing treatment contains natural antibiotic and antibacterial herbs.

> ½ teaspoon powdered goldenseal
> ¼ teaspoon powdered echinacea
> 6 drops tea tree essential oil
> Purified water

Combine the ingredients with enough water to form a paste. Apply to the affected area. Leave on the skin for at least 20 minutes, allowing the mixture to dry. Rinse with tepid water.

✺ Smart Shopping ✺

In 1996 alone, cosmetics manufacturers launched more than seventeen hundred new skin care products. Cleansers, scrubs, moisturizers, antiaging formulas, and even cellular renewal creams . . . each one supposedly better than the rest. Yet, 90 percent of the ingredients in these commercially available "miracle" creams and lotions are made in a chemist's lab.

Can you avoid synthetic chemicals and still have the convenience of shopping off-the-shelf? Yes! To get you started, here is a listing of nontoxic products that can actually nourish your skin.

Cleansers

Manufacturer	Product
Abra Therapeutics	Detox Complexion Wash
Annemarie Börlind	LL Cleansing Lotion
Aubrey Organics	Blue Green Algae Cleansing Cream
	Mandarin Magic Facial Cleanser
	Rosa Mosqueta Rose Hip Complexion Soap
	Seasoap Cleansing Cream
Beeswork	Nature's Cleanser
Botanics of California	Chamomile Cleanser
Compliments of Nature	Pure and Organic Skin Cleanser
Dr. Hauschka	Cleansing Milk
	Cleansing Cream
Jakaré	Liquid Glycerine Cleanser
	Refreshing Cleanser
Lily of Colorado	Lily Cleanser
	Lily Seaweed Cleanser
NaturElle	Facial Cleansing Gelee
Neways	Milky Cleanser
	TLC Cleansing Lotion
Paul Penders	Calendula Comfrey Cleansing Milk
	Peppermint Juniper Cleansing Gel
	Rosemary Elderflower Cleansing Milk
Perfectly Beautiful	Radiant Skin Cleanser

Scrubs

Manufacturer	Product
Aubrey Organics	Jojoba Meal and Oatmeal Facial Scrub
Botanics of California	Mint Exfoliator
Burt's Bees	Farmer's Market Citrus Facial Scrub
Jakaré	Purifying Scrub
Penny Island	Gentle Oat and Honey Facial Scrub

Toners and Astringents

Manufacturer	Product
Aubrey Organics	Green Tea Toner
	Herbal Facial Astringent
	Rosa Mosqueta Lavender Facial Toner
Beeswork	Nature's Toner
Botanics of California	Rosemary Toner
Burt's Bees	Farmer's Market Apple Cider Vinegar Toner
Dr. Hauschka	Clarifying Toner
Lily of Colorado	Lily Herbal Astringent

Moisturizers

Manufacturer	Product
Aubrey Organics	Blue Green Algae Antioxidant Moisturizer
	Rejeunesse Moisturizing Cream
	Vegecol TCM
Beeswork	Fabuleux Visage Face Cream
Botanics of California	Linden Flower Moisturizer
Burt's Bees	Moisturizing Cream
Dr. Hauschka	Moisturizing Day Cream
Jakaré	Revitalizing Face Treatment
Lily of Colorado	Facial Lotion
	Lily Moisturizing Cream
Neways	Skin Enhancer
Penny Island	Hydrating Facial Moisturizer
Perfectly Beautiful	Hydration
	Radiant Moisture Therapy

Facial Mists

Manufacturer	Product
Aubrey Organics	Sparkling Mineral Water Herbal Mist
Burt's Bees	Burt's Complexion Mist
	Farmer's Market Mist with Carrot Seed Oil
Jakaré	Renewing Mist
Neways	Bio-Mist Activator

Facial Masks

Manufacturer	Product
Aubrey Organics	Blue Green Algae Herbal Antioxidant Mask
	Rosa Mosqueta Mask
	Seaclay
Aztec Secret	Indian Healing Clay
Botanics of California	Meadowsweet Clay Mask
Burt's Bees	Green Goddess Clay Mask
Dr. Hauschka	Face Mask
Jakaré	Clarifying Clay Mask
Lily of Colorado	Botanical Enzyme Exfoliant Mask
Paul Penders	Mix and Mask
	Peppermint Arnica Beauty Mask
Penny Island	Papaya and Honey Facial Mask

Facial Steam Baths

Manufacturer	Product
Aubrey Organics	Face Flowers
Burt's Bees	Green Goddess Facial Sauna
Dr. Hauschka	Facial Steam Bath
Jakaré	Flower and Herb Steaming Blend

Night Creams

Manufacturer	Product
Aubrey Organics	Vegetarian Rejuvenation
Botanics of California	Evening Primrose Night Cream
Burt's Bees	Beeswax and Bee Pollen Night Cream
Dr. Hauschka	Skin Conditioner "N"
Jakaré	Enriching Face Treatment
Lily of Colorado	Lily Lotion
Paul Penders	Avocado Ginseng Night Cream
	Wheatgerm Honeysuckle Night Cream
Penny Island	Nourishing Facial Cream

Acne Treatments

Manufacturer	Product
Jakaré	Active Remedy
Paul Penders	Blemish Away
Perfectly Beautiful	Radiant Blemish Treatment

Eye Treatments

Manufacturer	Product
Botanics of California	Immortelle Emollient Eye Cream
Burt's Bees	Beeswax and Royal Jelly Eye Creme
	Bright Eyes Tea Bags
Dr. Hauschka	Eye Lid Cream
Jakaré	Aloe Eye Treatment/Make-up Remover
	Nourishing Eye Treatment/Make-up Remover
Paul Penders	Carotene Eye Gelee
Perfectly Beautiful	Radiant Under Eye Treatment

Antiaging Treatments

Manufacturer	Product
Abra Therapeutics	Cellular Gold PhytoSerum
Beeswork	AHA Gel Mask
Jakaré	Essential Nutrients
Neways	Wrinkle Garde
Nonie of Beverly Hills	AHA!
Paul Penders	GlycoFruit Treatment
	Herbal Citrus Fruit Exfoliant

Sun Protection

Manufacturer	Product
Abra Therapeutics	Natural Mineral Sun Block SPF-18
Aubrey Organics	Green Tea Sunblock
	Saving Face Sun Spray SPF-15

	Titania SPF-25 Full Spectrum Sunblock
	Ultra Natural Herbal Sunblock SPF-15
Logona Kosmtik's	Sun Milk
Neways	Sunbrero

5

Godiva's Glory: Hair Care

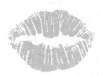

*"And forget not that the earth delights to feel your bare feet
and the winds long to play with your hair."*
—Kahlil Gibran

If the eyes are the window to the soul, then hair is the barometer of the body, reflecting our general health and well-being. Even though the hair we see is actually dead material, it can tell us a great deal about our physical condition. Dry, flaky hair can indicate nutritional deficiencies, especially shortages of essential fatty acids, zinc, and the B vitamins. Dull, lifeless hair can precede the symptoms of disease, and stress can result in breakage and even hair loss.

While we can't always control the inner forces affecting our tresses, we can fight the external war waged on our hair. Daily exposure to sun, wind, and pollution can result in hair that has lost its sheen and manageability. Blow-dryers, curling irons, and hot rollers rob hair of moisture and essential fatty acids. Frequent combing and brushing, especially when hair is wet, can damage the cuticle layer of the hair. The worst culprits, however, are the scores of chemical concoctions we apply to our hair every day.

Unlike natural hair care products that nourish the hair and scalp, petro-chemically based cleaners, conditioners, and styling aids can strip the hair of natural oils. If used regularly, these products can turn hair dull and dry, making it prone to split ends and breakage. Synthetic remedies, such as deep conditioners and hot oil treatments, just make matters worse.

But what about the damage you can't see?

Is Your Shampoo Killing You?

Of all the hair care products on the market today, shampoos are the products most often reported to the Food and Drug Administration (FDA) for causing adverse reactions.[1] Full of harsh detergents and synthetic fragrances, shampoos not only remove the natural oils from hair and scalp but also can be highly irritating, occasionally resulting in contact dermatitis. What's worse, common irritants such as polyethylene glycol, quaternium-15, 2-bromo-2-nitro-1,3-diol, and DMDM hydantoin can degrade into formaldehyde.

One of the most controversial irritants found in commercial shampoos is the surfactant sodium lauryl sulfate (SLS), also known as sodium laureth sulfate. Although often listed as being derived from coconuts, synthetic SLS is anything but natural. According to Ruth Winter, author of *A Consumer's Dictionary of Cosmetic Ingredients*, SLS is prepared by sulfation of lauryl alcohol, followed by neutralization with sodium carbonate, more commonly known as soda ash.[2]

Known in the industry as an aggressive cleaner, SLS is used by researchers to induce skin sensitivity in laboratory animals. This cytotoxic (cell-killing) chemical easily penetrates the skin, damaging and altering its structure and function.[3]

Another serious problem with SLS is its tendency to react with other ingredients to form the nitrosamine NDELA. Contamination from NDELA most commonly occurs when SLS is combined with diethanolamine or triethanolamine, abbreviated on product labels as DEA and TEA. "Lifelong use of these products clearly poses major avoidable cancer risks to the great majority of U.S. consumers, particularly infants and young children," warns Samuel S. Epstein, M.D., professor of environmental and occupational medicine at the University of Illinois School of Public Health and coauthor of *The Safe Shopper's Bible.*[4]

Although not all products containing SLS, DEA, and TEA are contaminated with nitrosamines, a great number of them are. In two surveys conducted in 1991, twenty-seven out of twenty-nine hair care products were found to be contaminated with high concentrations of NDELA. As a direct result of these surveys, the European Union took swift action to eliminate DEA from cosmetics and personal care products.[5] Yet, despite an explicit warning by the Cosmetics, Toiletry, and Fragrance Association concerning the dangers of NDELA contamination, the U.S. cosmetics industry continues to include DEA in most products. The FDA, which confirmed the findings of both surveys, is apparently siding with the manufacturers since it has yet to take any action to protect consumers from these carcinogenic impurities.[6]

More serious still, a recent study by the National Toxicology Program (NTP) found that these compounds may not need to interact with other chemicals to pose a potential health hazard. The study, released in December 1997, found that DEA *by itself* may have a stronger carcinogenic effect than when it's combined with other ingredients.[7] According to the NTP, repeated skin application of DEA and its fatty acid derivative, cocamide-DEA, was found to cause liver and kidney cancer in mice. The study also emphasized that DEA, when absorbed through the skin, accumulates in the organs, where it can induce long-term toxic effects.

The Condition of Your Conditioner

Standing on the Senate floor, longtime cosmetics safety advocate Senator Edward Kennedy recently told his peers of a six-year-old girl in Oakland, California, who suffered painful second-degree burns on her neck and ears after her mother applied an over-the-counter hair care product to her head. Another woman's hair caught fire as a result of her using a styling gel.[8] While we may think of conditioners and styling products as relatively benign, their use can result in both short- and long-term health problems. Burns, face and eye irritations, and hair loss are just a few of the complaints the FDA receives every year concerning over-the-counter conditioners and styling aids.

Most mainstream and many "natural" conditioners and cream rinses depend on synthetic petrochemicals to thicken hair, along with artificial colors and fragrances to make the product pleasant to use. That tangle-free, silky feel is usually a result of quaternary compounds and preservatives that are added to discourage bacteria. Another way manufacturers discourage the growth of microbes is with the addition of germicides, such as benzalkonium chloride. Last but not least, emulsifiers such as polysorbate 80, which may be contaminated with 1,4-dioxane, are added to keep the product from separating while it waits patiently on the store shelf for an uninformed consumer.

Setup for Disaster

A helmet of cementlike hair lacquer may not be the look you're after, but there are times when holding your hair in place is a necessity. Enter the vast array of setting lotions, styling gels, mousses, and hair sprays. But before you reach for your favorite styling product, consider this: along with the water and alcohol found in most setting lotions, styling gels, and mousses, most products contain not only TEA but also beta-naphthol—a coal tar derivative. Fatal poisonings have been reported from external applications of this chemical.[9] Add an antiseptic, such as creosol or phenol (better known as carbolic acid), and you have a toxic treatment ready to tame even the most stubborn locks.

Once you've got your hair looking the way you want it, do you reach for the hair spray to keep it that way? Available in aerosols and pumps, hair sprays deposit a coating of polyvinylpyrrolidone, or PVP, to the surface of your hair. If that sounds like something you'd use to build a sprinkler system, you're not far off. PVP is related to plastics and stiffens the hair to keep it in place. But along with coating your hair, the ingredients in hair spray also coat your respiratory tract, potentially leading to throat and lung irritations. Other ingredients often contained in hair spray include TEA, shellac, and PEG compounds.

While it's best to avoid using this type of product at all, if you must use one, do so in a well-ventilated area, and never use an aerosol hair spray. Aerosols create a greater health risk since the particles are considerably smaller and more readily inhaled. In fact, the Irish Medical Organisation considers them enough of a potential hazard that it has proposed a ban on aerosol sprays in communal changing rooms, such as school gyms.

A Color to Dye For

We love color, especially when it comes to our hair. But walking into most hair salons for a quick color change is like entering a toxic cloud of ammonia and formaldehyde, not to mention an alphabet soup of chemicals you can't smell. Over-the-counter hair dyes aren't much better, with most containing potential irritants and carcinogens. Since two out of every five American women dye their hair, it's important to know the risks involved. What's really in a box of Nice 'n Easy besides that handy pair of plastic gloves?

For starters, there's the controversial group of readily absorbed petroleum-based chemicals—coal tar derivatives. At least eight separate studies have indicated that women who dye their hair frequently are at a greater risk of developing hematopoietic cancers. A report published in the February 2, 1994, issue of the *Journal of the National Cancer Institute* showed that women who used black hair dye for more than twenty years have a higher risk of developing non-Hodgkin's lymphoma and multiple myeloma.[10] Another report, published in the October 15, 1993, issue of the *American Journal of Epidemiology*, stated that consumers who used permanent or semipermanent hair dyes for sixteen years or more had an increased risk of leukemia.[11] A separate study conducted by the Harvard School of Public Health and the University of Athens Medical School suggested that women who used hair dyes five times or more per year had twice the risk of developing ovarian cancer than women who had never used hair dyes.[12] With the potentially deadly long-term side effects associated with modern hair dyes, going gray doesn't seem so bad after all.

Another ingredient to avoid is phenylenediamine. Used as an intermediate in coal tar dyes, this chemical has been demonstrated to cause cancer in animals. A New York University study conducted in 1979 also linked phenylenediamine to breast cancer in humans,[13] although a recent study by the Fred Hutchinson Cancer Research Center in Seattle showed no correlation.[14]

In addition, products containing phenylenediamine compounds can cause blindness if the solution drips into the eyes. Never use any product that carries the following warning on the package:

CAUTION: This product contains ingredients that may cause skin irritation on certain individuals, and a preliminary test according to accompanying directions should first be made. This product must not be used for dyeing the eyelashes or eyebrows; to do so may cause blindness.

Immediate consequences can also lurk behind the promises of a vibrant new shade of hair color. Most such products are highly alkaline and have the potential of being extremely irritating. They may also result in severe and possibly deadly allergic reactions, as one fifty-nine-year-old woman discovered when she nearly died from an allergic reaction to her hair coloring.[15] Also, according to doctors at the University of Chicago Hospital's Department of Internal Medicine, a sixty-eight-year-old woman did succumb to fatal anaphylaxis as a result of her using a new hair dye.[16]

The Permanent Effects of Permanent Waves

Have you ever wished you could improve the hair Mother Nature gave you? Either it's too straight or it's too curly. Too thin or too thick. You're in luck! Through the magic of chemicals, you can painlessly change the structure of your hair with just one visit to the salon. Sound too good to be true? It is.

Cold-process permanent waves were first introduced in 1941 and have enjoyed enormous popularity ever since. However, while this process can give us what nature didn't, virtually all conventional perms contain serious toxins. Thioglycolic acid, the primary ingredient in chemical perms, works by swelling and penetrating the hair shaft, causing it to collapse and take on the shape of the rods used to "set" the hair. Once the hair is set, a neutralizing solution is applied *at just the right moment* to stop the process. Timing is key. Yet, more often than not, the thioglycolates are left on the hair too long. Not surprisingly, this damages and weakens hair. The result is overly processed hair that is more susceptible to ultraviolet and chemical damage. This damage is compounded by the surfactants commonly added to the processing solution to remove oil from the hair and scalp, increasing the penetration of the thioglycolates. Since perms remain on the hair and scalp for longer periods of time than most other treatments, absorption of these chemicals is greater.

Among the injuries reported to the FDA resulting from the use of permanent waves are skin and eye irritations, swelling of legs and feet, and swelling of the eyelids. These products are also suspected of causing low blood sugar. It's a high price to pay for a bit of curl and body.

On the other hand, if you're one of those people with too much curl, don't think you're without risk. Thioglycolic acid is also used in chemical hair straighteners. Highly alkaline, these solutions contain strong ingredients that can result in first- to third-degree burns and even hair loss. If that weren't enough, most chemical straighteners contain allergens and skin irritants such as polyethylene glycol, TEA, propylene glycol, and synthetic fragrance. At best, these products will dry out hair and cause it to become brittle.

Back to Basics

Hair is made up of almost pure protein, and although it is wonderfully strong and elastic, it can take only so much abuse from synthetic petrochemicals, curling irons, and blow-dryers. Returning your hair to its naturally beautiful state requires daily maintenance and the development of healthy habits. A hit-or-miss strategy can't make up for the daily practice of gentle care.

Before you can develop a healthy hair routine, you need to know what you're dealing with. Since every head of hair is different, evaluating your hair is the first step toward designing an individual hair care program that's right for you. First, consider your hair's texture. Is it thin and fine, or thick and coarse? Curly or straight? Next, to discover what type of hair you have, check Table 5.1 to find the description that most closely matches your own hair.

Table 5.1 ❧ What's Your Type?

Normal:	Normal hair is glossy, with good elasticity, and grows at a healthy rate. It's not fraught with tangles and split ends. The sebaceous glands produce just the right amount of oil to keep the hair healthy and balanced.
Dry:	Dull and brittle, dry hair suffers from numerous split ends. While some people don't produce enough natural oil to keep the hair and scalp lubricated, dry hair is usually the result of self-inflicted abuse—overexposure to sun and wind, heat from styling appliances, or too many chemical treatments.
Oily:	Thanks to overactive sebaceous glands, oily hair is often thought of as greasy, sometimes to the extent of appearing stringy. Weighed down by excess oil, it lacks the light, clean look of well-balanced hair. Unfortunately, people with oily hair often have accompanying skin problems, especially around the hairline.

Secrets of Healthy Hair

Shampooing is the first step toward healthy hair. How often you should shampoo depends on the type of hair you have. If your hair is excessively oily, you may want to shampoo daily. If you have dry or damaged hair, once a week may be right for you.

No matter how often you wash your hair, maximize your shampoo treatment by using a wide-tooth comb to untangle hair, starting at the ends and working up. Wet your hair thoroughly and then apply a small amount of shampoo, gently working it through the hair. Starting at the crown, work the lather down the length of your hair. Erratic, undirected motions only result in more tangles.

While healthy hair has a life span of two to six years, its birth begins at the root. Nourished by a network of blood vessels, the root is the only living part of the hair. It makes sense, then, to pay particular attention to the scalp, the place where life begins. Massaging the scalp while you shampoo is the single most important thing you can do for your hair. Using your fingertips, gently massage your scalp in a circular pattern for a minute or two. This simple act stimulates the scalp's rich blood supply and helps flush away metabolic waste.

If your hair is dry or badly damaged, use a good conditioner after every shampoo. Instead of reaching for a petrochemically based conditioner, treat your hair with a natural oil conditioner infused with herbs. Although there are several brands on the market, you can experiment with one of the formulas at the end of this chapter for a customized conditioner. To use, pour a small amount of conditioner into the palm of your hand, and then rub your hands together. Run your hands through your wet hair several times, working the conditioner from the scalp to the ends. After a minute or two, rinse thoroughly. Hair care experts recommend rinsing for several minutes to remove all traces of shampoo and conditioner. To add shine and restore the natural pH balance of your scalp, finish with a rinse of either diluted lemon juice (for blonds) or diluted apple cider vinegar (for brunettes and redheads).

How you dry your hair can also affect the health of your scalp. Resist the temptation to "scrub" hair dry. Instead, gently squeeze out the moisture in the folds of a thick towel. Once the excess moisture has been removed, air dry your hair whenever possible. Since blow-dryers rob hair of vital moisture, it's best to avoid them. If you must use a blow-dryer, purchase one with a "cool button." Alternate between "warm" and "cool," using the button with the lowest setting possible, and keep the air moving!

Although brushing your hair distributes the scalp's oil, the fabled one hundred strokes a night probably did more harm than good. If you must brush, never brush hair when it's wet—that's a surefire path to breakage and split ends. Instead, use a wide-tooth comb or, better yet, your fingers to gently detangle and shape. Also, instead of using a metal or plastic brush, opt for one made of natural bristles. A natural-bristle brush distributes the scalp's oil evenly, leaving your hair shiny and tangle-free. For combing the hair, buy a wooden comb with well-spaced teeth. Avoid combs with sharp, narrowly spaced metal or plastic teeth. Although inexpensive, this type of comb will tear hair, resulting in split ends.

How you wear your hair may be a reflection of your personality and lifestyle, but no hairstyle can mask unhealthy hair. If you wear your hair in an elaborate "do," you may want to explore a style that requires less maintenance. However you wear your hair, it pays to get regular trims, regardless of your hair's length. Split ends vanish, and you're left with a "finished" look.

Rx for Problem Hair

Although following a good hair care program can help keep hair and scalp healthy, there are times when stronger measures are required. At one time or another, we've all suffered from overexposure to the sun's burning rays, the occasional flake, or a few too many split ends. Luckily, there are measures you can take to prevent and correct these hair "emergencies."

Sun Damage

Whether or not you're the outdoor type, chances are your hair and scalp have occasionally been fried after a long day in the sun. What you can't see is the damage that too much sun has on your hair's delicate moisture balance. If you spend a lot of time outdoors, especially in summer, look for hair care products containing vitamin E, a natural sunscreen. Although these products help prevent damage, they don't offer absolute protection, so try to limit your exposure to early morning and late afternoon. If you must spend time in the sun between the hours of 11:00 A.M. and 2:00 P.M. (the hottest part of the day), cover up with a hat or scarf.

What if the damage is already done? To minimize the pain of a sunburned scalp, soak a cotton ball in apple cider vinegar or aloe vera juice, and gently dab it over the burned area. To prevent your scalp from peeling and flaking, use a shampoo containing alpha hydroxy acids.

Use a good conditioner for hair that is moderately burned, concentrating the product on the ends, where moisture loss is more pronounced. Badly burned hair may require a bit more help. To restore your hair's moisture balance, try an intensive hot oil treatment weekly until the problem is corrected.

Dandruff

Dandruff is an irregularity of the scalp's oil glands believed to be caused by a yeastlike fungus. The result is an itchy scalp and a nonstop downpour of tiny white flakes. Unfortunately, science hasn't come up with a foolproof cure for this irritating and often embarrassing condition. The best it can offer are dandruff shampoos containing zinc pyrithione, a bactericide and fungicide that reportedly damages the nerves, or selenium sulfide, a severe eye irritant that has been found to damage the liver in animal experiments.[17] If you're plagued by true dandruff, instead of reaching for the Head & Shoulders, rub your scalp with a cut clove of garlic before you shampoo. The antibiotic properties in the garlic discourage fungal growth. Follow your shampoo with a conditioner containing tea tree oil, or give yourself a deep conditioning treatment using plain yogurt. Gently massage the yogurt into your scalp, then cover with plastic wrap and a warm towel. Let the yogurt work for thirty minutes before thoroughly rinsing. Used on a regular basis, a yogurt treatment is said to control fungus and the resulting flakes.

What we often think of as dandruff is simply an overly dry scalp shedding small clumps of dead skin. This condition can be caused by harsh chemicals and overexposure to the elements, as well as stress, illness, and hormonal imbalances. In addition, some nutritionists believe that diet is often to blame. An excess of junk foods and saturated fats, combined with deficiencies in essential fatty acids, the B vitamins, and minerals such as zinc, can all contribute to the condition. If your diet is the cause of your dry scalp, forgo your trips to the Golden Arches and boost your intake of essential fatty acids such as flaxseed oil. To treat a dry, flaky scalp topically, try rinsing your hair with an infusion of thyme, chaparral, or burdock root.

Breakage

Breakage is usually the result of owner abuse and mishandling. A regular routine that includes excessive use of artificial heat and harsh chemicals is a guaranteed prescription for split ends. Since hair is dead material and doesn't have the ability to repair itself, the only real cure is to cut off the damage. While regular trims help control split ends, you can prevent breakage by following the hair care basics just described. To temporarily improve the appearance of your hair, use a raw-egg shampoo. The protein in the egg "glues" down the outer layer of hair, leaving you with a smooth look.

Fallout: The Problem of Hair Loss

Contrary to popular belief, hair loss isn't just a man's problem. While it's normal for a woman to lose fifty to one hundred hairs a day, it's estimated that nearly 20 million American women suffer from excessive hair loss. Unlike men, whose hair usually recedes into the familiar horseshoe shape, women often find their hair thinning at the crown. Although genetics is often blamed for hair loss, some researchers believe that the problem can be traced to an adverse reaction to topical chemicals, poor circulation, illness, stress, or even poor nutrition. Age is also a factor. By the age of forty, 25 percent of women begin to experience some hair loss. By the time women reach menopause, that figure jumps to 60 percent.

Over the last decade, researchers have made some headway in formulating chemical cures for hair loss. Originally used to treat prostate enlargement in men, finasteride (marketed under the brand name Propecia) has been found to reverse some types of hair loss. Approved by the FDA for use on men only, finasteride works by interfering with the hormone testosterone. But the side effects can be serious. Along with the occurrence of impotence in the men studied, researchers caution that use of the drug, even at a reduced dosage, may result in birth defects in male offspring.[18] Women in their reproductive years are warned not to take finasteride under any circumstances—*not even to touch the pills*, since handling may lead to absorption of the drug through the skin. Although finasteride is off-limits to women of childbearing age, proponents speculate that it may be approved for use by post-menopausal women in the near future. While there are no studies on the safety of long-term use in either men or women, some of the other side effects noted during the clinical trials included dizziness, headaches, loss of strength, abdominal pain, diarrhea, and difficulty urinating.

Another product approved by the FDA to treat hair loss is the familiar Rogaine, a topical minoxidil solution. Hailed by marketers as a miracle cure, Rogaine doesn't work for everyone, and the quality of regrowth is often poor.

Somewhat expensive ($20 to $30 a pop), the product needs to be applied twice a day, a less-than-convenient drawback. Moreover, if you stop using the product, growth stops too, so it's a long-term commitment once you begin treatment. Once available only by prescription, Rogaine in a 2 percent solution first hit the shelves several years ago as an over-the-counter remedy. Because of the product's popularity, a 5 percent solution, marketed by Pharmacia & Upjohn as Rogaine Extra Strength, was approved by the FDA for over-the-counter sales in 1997. Yet, a Hungarian study reported that using minoxidil can result in changes to the heart,[19] and the manufacturer cautions women who are pregnant, attempting pregnancy, or breast-feeding to avoid using the product.

Fortunately, there are some natural alternatives to preventing hair loss. If you don't already take a balanced vitamin B compound, start. Look for a brand that contains at least 300 micrograms (mcg) of biotin, since a deficiency of this particular B vitamin has been linked to hair loss. If you can't find a multivitamin containing biotin, supplement this critical vitamin with natural sources. Brown rice, bran, and soybeans are all good dietary sources of biotin. Also, avoid eating eggs, which can bind biotin and prevent its absorption into the body.

Although not scientifically proved, supplementing your daily diet with 500 milligrams (mg) each of L-cysteine and L-methionine is said to help prevent hair loss and improve the quality and texture of the hair you have. Drinking Kombucha tea is another remedy hailed by proponents to halt the loss of hair.

If you're losing hair because of poor circulation, massage your scalp daily to get the blood going. Use a stimulating essential oil, such as rosemary or lavender, to increase the effectiveness of the massage. Other herbs traditionally believed to stimulate and strengthen new growth include bay, birch, calendula, horsetail, nettle, and sage.

Table 5.2 lists the most helpful herbal remedies for hair problems.

Homemade Hair Care

Creating your own hair care products not only assures you of pure, natural ingredients but also allows you to customize the formulas to your own needs and desires. The formulas in this section are easy to make, and most keep well at room temperature.

Table 5.2 🍂 Herbal Remedies for Hair

Whether you buy your hair care products or make them yourself, familiarity with the healing properties of different herbs can help you tailor the products you use to your individual needs. Most of the herbs listed here are available in dried form or as essential oils.

If You Need . . .	Useful Herbs	Comments and Cautions
antiseptic/ antibacterial	calendula, eucalyptus, lavender, lemon, neroli,* pine, rosemary, sage, southernwood, tea tree oil*	If you are fair-haired, be aware that using sage as an antiseptic rinse on a regular basis can darken hair.
curl enhancer	rosemary	
dandruff prevention	bay leaf, lavender, lemon, neroli,* nettle, rosemary	
dry hair conditioner	aloe vera, burdock, kelp, lavender, nasturtium, rose, rose geranium, rosemary, sandalwood,* sesame,* sunflower*	
hair colorant	calendula, chamomile, elder, henna, nettle, sage, walnut	Used as a rinse, these herbs color hair gradually.
hair conditioner	birch, elder, henna, kelp, lavender, lemon, nettle, rosemary, sage, southern-wood	Clear henna should be used for conditioning.
hair loss preventive	calendula, kelp, lemon, nettle, parsnip, peach leaves, rosemary, sage, southernwood, willow, yarrow	
hair oil	almond,* burdock, elder, lavender, olive,* rosemary, sesame,* sunflower*	*continued*

If You Need . . .	Useful Herbs	Comments and Cautions
hair stimulant	bay leaf, birch, calendula, lavender, nettle, rosemary	
hair strengthener	horsetail, nettle, oat straw	These herbs are high in silica.
hair tonic	burdock, comfrey, elder, lavender, lemon, nettle, sage	
oily hair remedy	cedarwood,* lemon, lemongrass, patchouli,* sage	
rinse	chamomile, calendula, elder flowers, lavender, lemon, nettle, rosemary, sage	Use as a tea, or combine with apple cider vinegar to remove traces of dirt and shampoo.
scalp conditioner	burdock, chaparral, thyme	Use to treat a dry scalp.
setting lotion	calendula buds	Use as a tea before setting hair.
shampoo	lemon, nettle, rosemary, sage, soapbark, yarrow	

*Available in oil form only.

Shampoos

Healthy hair begins as clean hair. If you can't find a truly natural shampoo at your neighborhood health food store, try making your own. As effective as commercial varieties, homemade shampoos use a base of pure liquid castile soap. Note: Castile soap will leave a residue, which can be removed with one of the rinses described later in this chapter.

California Citrus Shampoo   YIELD: 8 ounces
Reminiscent of a day in the sun, this shampoo will bring out the highlights in your hair.

½ cup liquid castile soap
4 tablespoons fresh lemon juice
½ cup distilled water
5 drops neroli essential oil

Combine the ingredients and pour into a clean plastic bottle. Cap and store in a cool, dry spot for a day or two, shaking twice a day to thoroughly blend the ingredients.

Southwestern Shampoo   Yield: 10 ounces
Native Americans of the Southwest discovered the natural beauty benefits of jojoba, the oil-rich shrub so prevalent in the Sonoran Desert. This shampoo conditions as it cleans, helping to repair dry, damaged hair.

½ cup liquid castile soap
½ cup aloe vera juice
1 teaspoon jojoba oil
½ cup avocado oil

Mix the ingredients and pour into a plastic bottle with a tight-fitting lid. Since the ingredients will separate when left standing, shake well before every use.

Herbal Shampoo   Yield: 8 ounces
Nettles and horsetail have been used for centuries to strengthen and repair hair. Used regularly, this shampoo helps improve the condition of hair while adding shine and manageability.

1 tablespoon rosemary
2 teaspoons dried nettles
1 teaspoon dried horsetail
½ cup distilled water
½ cup liquid castile soap
10 drops lavender essential oil

Combine the rosemary, nettles, horsetail, and water in a small saucepan. Over medium heat, bring the mixture to a boil. Turn off the heat and let steep for 1 hour. Strain and cool. Add the soap and essential oil, stirring well to mix. Store in a plastic bottle with a tight-fitting lid.

Old-Fashioned Egg Shampoo
YIELD: 1 application

Restore softness and manageability to dry hair with this time-tested protein shampoo.

> 2 large eggs
> 3 tablespoons cider vinegar, or juice of half a lemon

Beat the eggs until frothy, and massage into scalp. Leave on for a few minutes before rinsing thoroughly with warm water. To cut the film left by the eggs, finish with a rinse of vinegar (for dark hair) or lemon juice (for light hair). Mix the vinegar or juice with 8 ounces of warm water. Pour through hair.

Dry Shampoo
YIELD: 1 application

When there's no time to wash your hair, try a dry shampoo to remove excess dirt and oil.

> ⅓ cup cornmeal
> 1 tablespoon arrowroot

Mix the ingredients. Standing over a sink, massage the mixture directly onto scalp and through hair. Wrap your head in a towel and allow the mixture to work for at least 15 minutes. To remove, brush hair gently until all of the residue is gone (do this over a sink or outside since the "fallout" can be quite messy).

Conditioners and Intensive Treatments

Dry, damaged, or overly processed hair can result in your hair looking more like a haystack than the crowning glory it was meant to be. The following conditioners are rich in natural oils that, when allowed to penetrate the hair, repair the damage done by sun, blow-dryers, and harsh chemicals. For especially damaged hair, use a good conditioner after every shampoo and a more intensive treatment once a week to restore moisture and manageability.

Instant Suds Softener
YIELD: 1 application

Beer adds manageability and shine to dull, lifeless hair.

> 1 cup warm beer

After shampooing, pour beer over hair, massaging it into your hair for a minute or two. Rinse well with warm water.

Mayonnaise Magic   YIELD: 1 application

An old standby, mayonnaise is still the best conditioner around for normal to dry hair. Add a bit of ginseng to boost flexibility and sheen.

1 cup good-quality mayonnaise
½ teaspoon powdered ginseng

Using a wire whisk, combine the ingredients in a small bowl until smooth. Massage into hair, working from the crown to the ends. Run your fingers through your hair several times to make sure each strand is coated. Cover with a plastic bag or shower cap, and relax for 15 minutes. Rinse thoroughly with warm water.

Dry-Scalp Conditioner   YIELD: 1 application

It's believed that yogurt and rosemary contain properties that moisturize the scalp and help control dandruff.

1 cup plain yogurt
5 drops rosemary essential oil

Using a wire whisk, combine the ingredients. Massage through hair, paying extra attention to your scalp. Cover with a plastic bag or shower cap. After 30 minutes, rinse thoroughly with warm water.

Pre-Sun Slicker   YIELD: 1 application

Try this rich conditioner before going out for a day in the sun, to prevent sun-damaged hair.

1 tablespoon crushed sage
1 tablespoon crushed nettles
½ cup avocado oil
½ cup jojoba oil
3 capsules vitamin E

Mix the ingredients together, and then slather the mixture through your hair. Using a wide-tooth comb, slick hair back until it is smooth and sleek. Thoroughly shampoo after sunning.

Deep-Conditioning Henna Treatment   YIELD: 1 application

Henna wraps each strand of hair with a protective coating, making it appear fuller. This coating also reflects light, making your hair shiny and radiant. Make sure you use wooden or plastic utensils to mix the henna since metal can cause an adverse reaction. Another word of caution: Don't use henna if your hair has been chemically treated. Henna can react with the chemicals already absorbed by your hair and leave you with unintended results.

½ cup distilled water
¼ cup colorless henna
2 teaspoons honey
Lavender or rosemary essential oil (optional)

Bring the water to a boil. Pour the henna into a separate bowl. Add the boiling water and honey and mix well. For extra conditioning, add a few drops of lavender or rosemary essential oil. Let the henna mixture sit for a few minutes to thicken, and then work into your hair, making sure each strand is coated. Wrap your hair in plastic, and cover with a warm towel. Let the henna work for 45 minutes to an hour before thoroughly rinsing. Follow with a shampoo that has a pH of 4.5 to 5.5. Dry and style as usual.

Intensive Jojoba Oil Conditioning Treatment   Yield: 1 application
An excellent treatment for badly damaged hair.

¼ cup jojoba oil
¼ cup sesame oil
1 tablespoon aloe vera gel
10 drops rosemary essential oil
5 drops rose geranium essential oil

Combine the jojoba and sesame oil in a small saucepan, and warm over medium heat. Add the aloe vera gel and stir until dissolved. Remove from heat, and add the rosemary and rose geranium essential oils. Work through hair, making sure it is saturated completely. Wrap your hair in plastic, and cover with a warm towel. Allow the mixture to work for 30 minutes. Follow with a shampoo.

Rinses

Used after shampooing, these rinses whisk away any traces of remaining dirt and shampoo, leaving you with incredibly clean hair. The herbs they contain also make these rinses healing tonics. To use any of the rinses listed here, simply pour a cupful over your head after you've shampooed and conditioned your hair. Unless otherwise specified, these formulas make enough rinse for fourteen applications.

Hair-Strengthening Rinse   YIELD: 80 ounces

High in silica, the herbs in this rinse strengthen weak or damaged hair. To enhance their strengthening ability, supplement the rinse by drinking a daily cup of horsetail tea.

> ½ gallon distilled water
> ¼ cup dried horsetail, cut coarsely
> ¼ cup dried nettles, cut coarsely
> ¼ cup dried oat straw, cut coarsely
> 2 cups apple cider vinegar

Pour the water into a large pot and bring to a boil. Using a square of cheesecloth or a large tea ball, secure the horsetail, nettles, and oat straw. Add them to the boiling water, cover, and reduce heat. Simmer for 10 to 15 minutes, and remove from heat. When cool to the touch, remove the herbs, and pour the liquid into a large plastic jug with a tight-fitting lid. Add the vinegar. Cap and shake to mix.

Nasturtium Hair Rinse   YIELD: 66 ounces

A lovely rinse for blond hair, nasturtium stimulates the root of the hair, promoting new growth.

> 1 cup nasturtium leaves, crushed
> ⅓ cup nasturtium flowers
> 1 1-inch slice fresh ginger, chopped
> ½ gallon distilled water
> ¼ cup freshly squeezed lemon juice

Place the nasturtium leaves and flowers, along with the chopped ginger, in a large bowl. Bring the water to a rapid boil. Immediately pour the boiling water over the herbs, and allow to steep for 30 minutes. Add the lemon juice and set aside to cool. When cool, pour into a large plastic jug with a tight-fitting lid.

Herbal Hair Tonic—Two Ways   YIELD: 72 ounces

A refreshing rinse packed with hair-healthy herbs. Adjust the ingredients to match your hair type.

Oily Formula	*Normal to Dry Formula*
¼ cup lemongrass	¼ cup lavender buds
2 tablespoons chamomile flowers	2 tablespoons rose petals
1 tablespoon oat straw	1 tablespoon nettles
½ gallon distilled water	½ gallon distilled water
1 cup lemon juice	2 cups cider vinegar
10 drops patchouli oil	10 drops rose oil

Wrap the herbs (first three ingredients) in a square of cheesecloth and secure with a rubber band. In a large pot, bring the water to a rapid boil. Turn off the heat and add the packet of herbs. Steep for 10 minutes. Remove the herbs and discard. Add the lemon juice or vinegar, and stir to mix. When cool, add the essential oil and mix thoroughly. Pour into a large plastic jug with a tight-fitting lid.

Tipsy Rosemary Rinse   YIELD: 1 application
This rinse acts as a gentle exfoliant. Full of alpha hydroxy acids, it's a perfect remedy if your scalp is sunburned or excessively dry and flaky.

    1 cup red wine
    5 drops rosemary essential oil

In a small, heavy-bottom saucepan, gently heat the wine until just barely warm. Remove from heat and add the rosemary essential oil. Massage into your scalp for a minute or two before rinsing thoroughly.

Clarifying Dandruff Rinse   YIELD: 1 application
The antiseptic and healing herbs in this rinse kill the fungus that causes dandruff.

    1 cup distilled water
    2 tablespoons apple cider vinegar
    10 drops lavender essential oil
    5 drops rosemary essential oil
    3 drops tea tree oil

In a small, heavy-bottom saucepan, slightly heat the water (110°F). Combine the vinegar, lavender essential oil, rosemary essential oil, and tea tree oil in a large plastic cup. Add the warmed water and stir to mix. Massage into your scalp for a minute or two before rinsing thoroughly.

Styling Aids

Unruly hair needn't be tamed with heavy waxes and petroleum products. Botanicals can help coax hair into shape while nourishing your hair and scalp.

Rosemary Hair Oil   YIELD: 4 ounces
To subdue frizz and flyaway hair, try a bit of this moisturizing oil.

  1 teaspoon rosemary
  ½ cup sunflower oil

Place the rosemary in a square of cheesecloth and secure. Place the packet of rosemary in a ceramic coffee mug. In a small, heavy-bottom saucepan, gently heat the oil until almost simmering. Remove from heat and pour over the rosemary. Allow to cool. Remove the packet, and pour the liquid into a small decorative glass bottle with a tight-fitting lid. To use, rub a few drops of oil in the palms of your hands. Smooth hands over hair.

Almond Styling Gel   YIELD: 8 ounces
If your hair needs a bit of extra body, try this fragrant styling gel.

  1 cup distilled water, warmed
  1 tablespoon agar
  1 teaspoon glycerin
  1 tablespoon almond oil
  4 drops almond extract

Combine the water and agar in a glass bowl, stirring until the agar is completely dissolved. Add the glycerin, almond oil, and extract, blending thoroughly. Refrigerate for 1 hour or until almost set. Remove the bowl from the refrigerator. Stir well and transfer into a glass or plastic container with a tight-fitting lid. Refrigerate for another hour. Stir the mixture once again before storing it at room temperature. This gel can be used on either wet or dry hair.

Calendula Styling Gel   YIELD: 8 ounces
For extra hold, this gel can't be beat. The sugar and protein combine with the calendula for an all-natural method of holding hair in place.

  1 tablespoon calendula buds
  1 cup distilled water

1 teaspoon agar
½ teaspoon granulated sugar

Place the calendula buds in a small glass bowl. Bring the water to a boil and pour over the buds. Steep for 15 minutes. Strain, returning the liquid to the bowl. Sprinkle the agar and sugar over the top, and stir to dissolve. Refrigerate until firm. Store in a glass or plastic jar with a tight-fitting lid.

Rosemary Mist   YIELD: 8 ounces

If you live in a dry climate or spend a lot of time in the sun, this mist can be a lifesaver. Give your hair a spritz periodically throughout the day to add moisture. The bonus? The rosemary enhances curl and body!

1 cup distilled water
1 tablespoon rosemary

Combine the water and rosemary in a small, heavy-bottom saucepan. Bring to a boil, and remove from heat. When the mixture has cooled, strain and store in a clean spritzer bottle.

Citrus-Herbal Hair Spray   YIELD: 8 ounces

The natural sugars in this deliciously scented hair spray help hold flyaway hair in place.

1 cup distilled water
1 1-inch piece tangerine peel
1 1-inch piece lemon peel
1 tablespoon grapefruit juice
2 drops neroli essential oil

In a small, heavy-bottom saucepan, bring the water to a boil. Place the tangerine and lemon peel in a small glass bowl. Pour the boiling water over the peel. Cover and allow to sit overnight. Strain the peel out of the bowl, and add the grapefruit juice and essential oil. Stir to blend thoroughly. Pour the solution into a clean spritzer bottle.

Sweet Lavender Hair Spray   YIELD: 8 ounces

This fragrant spray not only holds hair in place but also provides extra body.

    1 teaspoon granulated sugar
    1 cup distilled water, slightly warmed
    5 drops lavender essential oil

Dissolve the sugar in the water. Add the essential oil and stir well to mix. Pour into a clean spritzer bottle.

Hair Color

Whether we want a whole new look or simply need to hide a few gray hairs, nature can provide the color we crave. Exalted in ancient Indian literature and reportedly used by Cleopatra, henna has been used for centuries to color and condition. Today, henna is combined with other plant pigments, such as chamomile or walnut shells, to achieve different hues. Easy to use, henna powder is available in most health food stores.

Color can also come from a variety of other natural sources. Beets or cranberries provide a burnished red tint. Various shades of brown can be obtained from walnuts, pecans, coffee, or tea. And chamomile, marigolds, or dandelions will give blonds a golden glow. The only requirement for these plant dyes is that you begin with a base light enough to "take" the color.

Henna Hair Coloring   Yield: 1 application

Henna not only colors your hair but also transforms it into a radiant halo, reflecting light from the sun. Be sure to use wooden or plastic bowls and utensils since metal can react with the henna to give you unexpected results. Note: Never use henna on hair that has been chemically treated.

The following formula is for short to medium-length hair. For longer hair, simply double the amounts of henna and liquid.

    ¼ cup henna (any shade)
    ⅓ cup boiling distilled water or tea (see following instructions)

Place the henna in a small glass or plastic bowl. Add the boiling liquid, and mix thoroughly until you achieve a creamy consistency. Substituting tea (or coffee) for the water can enhance the final results. For example, black Ceylon tea will bring out golden highlights, and a strong chamomile tea will brighten blond hair; coffee will amplify brown tones. Allow the mixture to thicken for a few minutes before applying to clean, dry hair.

To apply, divide the hair into 1-inch sections. Beginning at the scalp, work the mixture evenly into each section. When all the hair is coated, cover hair with a plastic bag or plastic wrap. The henna should be allowed to work for 30 to 60 minutes, depending on the shade desired. Rinse out thoroughly, followed by a pH 4.5 to 5.5 shampoo. Dry and style as usual.

To create even more dramatic effects, add one of the following ingredients to your henna preparation:

For Extra Conditioning	1 egg, or 2 tablespoons plain yogurt
To Boost Brown or Red Tones	1 teaspoon ground ginger, allspice, or nutmeg
To Help Hold Color on Gray Hair	2 tablespoons apple cider vinegar
To Lighten Blond Hair	2 tablespoons lemon juice
To Add Fragrance	5 drops of your favorite essential oil

Nutty and Natural Hair Dye   YIELD: 2 ounces

Although the activity is labor intensive, various shades of brown can be obtained from the shells of nuts.

   1 dozen pecan or walnut shells
   ¼ cup distilled water

In a heavy-bottom frying pan, roast the nutshells until burned. When the shells have cooled, grind them as finely as possible (a coffee or spice grinder works well). Mix the powdered shells with enough distilled water to form a paste. Spread on hair, and cover with a plastic bag or wrap. Allow the mixture to work for 15 minutes to 1 hour, depending on desired results. Rinse out thoroughly, followed by a pH 4.5 to 5.5 shampoo. Dry and style as usual.

Botanical Tints   YIELD: 8 ounces

Let nature wash your hair with fresh new color. Although flowers, stems, leaves, bark, and seeds don't actually change the color of your hair, they impart a wonderful tint. To help guarantee the final outcome, do a strand test before applying the dye to your whole head. Check the strand periodically to calculate the time required to achieve the desired result.

3 cups plant material (see following instructions)
4 cups distilled water

Place the plant material in the bottom of a large saucepan or Dutch oven. Cover with the water and bring to a boil. Boil for 1 hour, and then strain. Return the liquid to the pan and boil for an additional hour. Cool before applying to hair. Wearing plastic gloves, pour the solution through hair. Cover with a plastic bag or wrap, and allow to work for 15 minutes to an hour, depending on the desired results. Rinse out thoroughly, followed by a pH 4.5 to 5.5 shampoo. Dry and style as usual.

To help decide which botanical is best for you, check the following chart.

Effect Desired	*Botanical Used*	*Part of Plant Used*
for blond hair	chamomile, dandelion	flowers
	onion	skin
for red hair	beets, cranberries	fruit
for brown hair	marigold	flowers
	cinnamon	bark
	acorn	nuts
	tobacco	leaves
	coffee	beans

❧ Smart Shopping ☙

Standing in the personal care and beauty section of your neighborhood health food store can be an overwhelming experience. An extraordinary number of "natural" hair care products line the shelves. How do you choose? While they all are likely to contain some natural ingredients, most aren't chemical-free. In fact, a surprising number of "natural" shampoos, conditioners, and styling products contain synthetic petrochemicals, which harm not only you but the earth as well.

Just a reminder: *read the label!* Particularly avoid products containing DEA, TEA, MEA, sodium lauryl sulfate, sodium laureth sulfate, and phenylenediamine.

To help you navigate the maze of commercial products on the market today, here are some that are actually good for your hair.

Shampoos

Manufacturer	Product
Aubrey Organics	Blue Green Algae Shampoo
	Camomile Shampoo
	Egyptian Henna Shampoo
	Green Tea Shampoo
	Honeysuckle Rose Shampoo
	Island Naturals Shampoo
	JAY Shampoo
	Primrose and Lavender Shampoo
	Rosa Mosqueta Shampoo
	White Camellia and Jasmine Shampoo
Bindi	Hair Wash
Dr. Hauschka	Shampoo
Earth Science	Hair Treatment Shampoo
	Herbal Astringent Shampoo
Ecco Bella	Dandruff Therapy Shampoo
	Wake-Me-Up Shampoo
Faith in Nature	Aloe Vera Shampoo
	Jojoba Shampoo
	Rosemary Shampoo
	Seaweed Shampoo
Giovanni	50/50 Balanced Shampoo
Jakaré	Conditioning Shampoo Bar
Mera	Shampoo for Dry Hair
	Shampoo for Normal Hair
	Shampoo for Oily Hair
Neways	Silken Mild Family Shampoo
Perfectly Beautiful	Radiant Hair Shampoo
Urtekram	Camomile Shampoo
	Desert Moments Shampoo
	Gypsy Night Dream Shampoo
	Ocean Mist Shampoo

Rose and Jasmine Shampoo
Soft Highlights

Conditioners

Manufacturer	Product
Aubrey Organics	Blue Green Algae Cream Rinse
	Green Tea Herbal Cream Rinse
	Honeysuckle Rose Conditioner
	Island Naturals Cream Rinse
	Primrose Tangle-Go
	Rosa Mosqueta Rose Hip Conditioner
	Rosemary and Sage Hair Rinse
	White Camellia and Jasmine Conditioner
Biopure	Apple with Pectin Conditioner
Burt's Bees	Farmer's Market Avocado Butter
Dr. Hauschka	Herbal Hair Conditioner
	Neem Hair Lotion
	Neem Hair Oil
Earth Preserv	Hair Vitalizer
Earth Science	Citresoft Conditioner
	Fragrance Free Conditioner
	Intensicare Conditioner
	Herbal Astringent Conditioner
Faith in Nature	Aloe Vera Conditioner
	Seaweed Conditioner
Giovanni	Direct Stay-In Conditioner
	Tea Tree Triple Treat Conditioner
Golden Lotus	Rosemary and Lavender Conditioner
Infinity	Camomile Conditioning Rinse
	Rosemary Conditioning Rinse
Jakaré	Conditioning Hair and Scalp Rinse
	Conditioning Hair Treatment
	Conditioning Scalp Treatment
Mera	Conditioner for Normal Hair
	Conditioner for Oily Hair
Neways	Exuberance Conditioner
Perfectly Beautiful	Radiant Hair Conditioner

Styling Aids

Manufacturer	Product
Aubrey Organics	B5 Design Gel
	Natural Missst Hairspray
Earth Science	Silk Forte Hair Styling Mist
	Silk Lite Hair Styling Mist
Honeybee Gardens	Wheat Therapy Hair Spray
Mera	Hair Spray
	Misting Gel
Naturade	Hair Spray with Jojoba
	Nonalcohol Styling Spray
Neways	Finishing Touch Hair Spray
	Replenishing Mist
	Sassy Spritz
Paul Penders	Hair Spritzer
Weleda	Rosemary Hair Oil

Hair Coloring

Manufacturer	Product
Igora Botanic	Hair Color
Light Mountain	Pure Henna
Rainbow Research	Pure Henna
VitaWave	Hair Color

Permanent Waves

Manufacturer	Product
VitaWave	Permanent Wave

6

Fingertips and Footnotes: Hand and Foot Care

"Morning stirs the feet and hands."

—T. S. Eliot

Nothing is more graceful or speaks more eloquently about how we care for ourselves than perfectly manicured hands and feet. Our hands can heal the sick and comfort those in need. They can express our creativity and emphasize our speech. Whatever our vocation—a concert pianist, a computer programmer, a factory worker, a new mother—our hands are the tools we use to accomplish our life's work. Made up of twenty-seven bones and a complex network of muscles, tendons, and nerves, these mechanical wonders also give us our first lessons about the world through our sense of touch.

But despite the importance of our hands, too often we ignore or, even worse, abuse them. We dash about bare-handed, exposing our hands to the sun, snow, and wind, which can dry them and leave them red, chapped, and flaky. If that weren't enough, the activities in which we engage every day can undermine beautiful hands and nails by subjecting them to harsh chemicals and detergents.

Carrying us through life's journey, our feet are our foundation. These biological masterpieces contain twenty-six bones, twenty-two joints, and a network of more than a hundred tendons, muscles, and ligaments, making it possible for us to walk, run, jump, and dance. In fact, according to the American Podiatric Medical Association (APMA), our feet carry us an average of seventy-five thousand miles by the time we are fifty,[1] quite possibly making them the hardest-working part of our body.

Yet, we rarely think of our feet unless they hurt. And hurt they will. Years of neglect can result in dry, rough skin and calluses. Ill-fitting shoes can lead to problems ranging from minor corns to structural deformities such as hammertoes and bunions. Even age can undermine your feet. As we get older, the fatty pads that cushion our feet gradually degenerate, reducing their ability to absorb shock. Once we pass the middle-age mark, this degeneration accelerates, particularly under the ball of the foot.

The upside is that much of the damage our hands and feet endure can be prevented with regular care. Using the gifts of nature instead of chemically packed cosmetics can help you rediscover the soft hands and silky feet you were born with.

Clean and Mean

Although keeping your hands clean is vital to healthy living, hand washing with soap can severely deplete the moisture from your skin. Made from a combination of fats and an alkali such as lye, traditional soap strips the skin of its natural oils. But these modern moisture thieves don't simply dry the skin. Today's soaps have redefined hand washing with myriad questionable ingredients.

Since soap isn't regulated by the Food and Drug Administration (FDA), many manufacturers add synthetic moisturizers and emollients such as petrolatum or mineral oil. These petroleum-based ingredients may leave the skin feeling soft right after use, but in the long run they can clog pores and actually pull moisture from the skin. What's more, many are common allergens and suspected carcinogens. For a natural alternative, try a pure glycerin soap. Made from the emollient-rich by-products of traditional soap manufacturing, these lovely transparent bars are more moisturizing than ordinary soap.

Other popular drugstore cleaners are designed to keep users germ-free, particularly the trendy new antibacterial soaps and waterless hand sanitizers. According to advertisers, cleanliness-conscious consumers can banish microscopic bugs wherever they lurk with these specially formulated soaps, particularly on their hands. Killing germs has become big business, with sales of about $1 billion in 2000 alone.[2] Because antibacterials are so profitable, almost half of all soaps currently on the market contain some type of bug-busting compound. Yet, at least one of the critter-killing ingredients found in these products, phenol-based dichloro-m-xylenol, may cause reproductive damage. Animal studies suggest that phenol may damage chromosomes and can lead to low birth weights in newborns.[3]

Some infectious disease experts are also very concerned that the overuse of antibacterial soaps and cleansers could kill beneficial bacteria and create drug-resistant strains of harmful bugs.[4] They cite the recent discovery of drug-resistant strains of bacteria that have occurred because of the overuse and misuse of antibiotics. Backing up their claim is a study by researchers at Tufts University School of Medicine in Boston, which found that triclosan, the most popular antibacterial ingredient, targets a specific bacterial gene instead of acting as a general, nonspecific biocide, giving this antibacterial chemical the potential for developing a resistant "super bug."[5] "Perhaps more dangerous," says Pat Costner, a senior scientist for Greenpeace, "is that one of the by-products of triclosan is dioxin."[6]

Triclosan is actually a derivative of 2,4-dichlorophenoxyacetic acid, more commonly known as the pesticide 2,4-D. In animal testing, 2,4-D has been found to be toxic to the blood, liver, and kidneys.[7] Triclosan is a prevalent contaminant in the environment, and Costner also notes that a Swedish study recently found high levels of this bactericide in human breast milk.[8]

The Moisture Game

Keeping our hands soft and smooth with a daily dose of moisturizing cream or hand lotion has always been the prescription for avoiding the problems associated with excessively dry skin. Without replenishing the moisture lost during our daily activities, our hands become subject to cracks and fissures, which can play host to germs and bacteria. What's more, chronic dryness thickens the skin, making it less able to absorb moisture. But will any hand lotion do? Can these modern moisturizing miracles really hydrate, even heal, parched hands?

The hand creams and lotions you see on drugstore shelves are often simply thicker versions of facial moisturizers and contain many of the same ingredients. Although these ingredients do make skin look and feel softer and smoother right after you use them, unlike plant-based emollients, it's doubtful whether they do anything but temporarily glue down dry, flaky skin cells with oil. And while they do help the skin hold water, they can also block pores, preventing the natural release of toxins.

Another emollient often found in hand lotions is lanolin. Although natural in origin, commercial lanolin can be contaminated with DDT and other carcinogenic substances.[9] Indeed, a toxicologic sampling of lanolin found that this widely used emollient contained sixteen pesticides, including diazinon, lindane, and dieldrin, persistent chlorine-based pesticides that are probable human carcinogens. Aware of the study, the FDA issued an alert warning manufacturers of the problem but noting that, in the agency's opinion, the levels found did not pose a health risk.[10]

Since hand lotions are basically a mixture of water and oil, emulsifiers are required to keep the product from separating. The most common emulsifier in hand lotions are PEGs, which may be contaminated with the volatile carcinogen dioxane. Triethanolamine (TEA) is also added as a dispersing agent and detergent. Tests at the University of Bologna in Italy have found TEA to be the most frequent sensitizer of any emulsifying agent.[11] Another study by the Aberdeen Royal Hospital Trust in Fostesterhill, United Kingdom, found that the risk of developing contact dermatitis rises when TEA is combined with stearic acid, another common additive in hand lotions.[12]

Last, but certainly not least, are the preservatives added to bolster the products' longevity. Common preservatives in mainstream moisturizers include formaldehyde-releasing DMDM hydantoin and quaternium-15, as well as potentially hormone-disrupting butyl-, ethyl-, methyl-, or propyl-parabens. Parabens have also been shown to have a greater potential for causing allergic reactions and contact dermatitis.

Moisture Moxie

Although dry weather can wick moisture away from the hands, the worst enemy is plain old water. Each time we expose our hands to water, particularly hot water, we lose moisture. If you've ever lounged in a nice hot bath for longer than you should, you've probably noticed that the tips of your fingers begin to resemble prunes. That's the visible sign of moisture loss. When you combine harsh detergents and cleaning solutions with hot water, you invite irritation and chapping.

Although most of us have experienced the effects of water-induced dryness firsthand, other activities also can instantly deplete moisture. Gardening is a prime culprit since soil can draw moisture out of your skin. But you don't have to get dirty to sabotage your hands. If you work in an office with reams of paper, you may have noticed how dry your palms and fingertips become by the end of the day. Surprisingly, ordinary paper can act as a blotter, sapping the moisture and protective oils from your hands. To guard against daily moisture loss, get into the habit of applying a good hand cream or lotion several times a day, particularly after your hands have been exposed to water.

Fortunately, you don't need to resort to chemical-filled creams and lotions to keep hands soft and supple. An array of chemical-free products on the market will help your skin retain moisture by providing a temporary barrier between you and the environment. Based on emollient-rich herbs and plant oils, these products don't simply coat the skin; they are absorbed into the skin, where they counteract dryness and promote healthy hands. To apply a natural hand lotion, pour a generous amount into your palm. Massage the lotion into the skin, concentrating on particularly dry or rough spots, until the lotion has been thoroughly absorbed.

Elemental Protection

As we rush from task to task, we rarely give any thought to how our daily activities impact the health of our hands until we notice painful dryness, flakiness, or even cracks. As we've seen, even ordinary things can dehydrate our hands. Since our hands are our tools for life, it's important to treat them with kindness each day.

Once upon a time, a lady would never dream of venturing out of the house without a pair of pristine white gloves. It was a symbol of social status, wealth, and breeding. It was also a way to protect delicate hands that never encountered a sink full of dirty dishes or a garden full of weeds. While the days of ladies in gloves have given way to women leading more productive, satisfying lives, gloves can still protect our hands from environmental damage.

Although our hands produce their own protective coating—a natural moisturizer made of sebum and water—hot water, detergents, and solvents remove this natural protection, leaving our hands vulnerable to dehydration. Donning a pair of rubber or latex gloves can offer protection from damage that can chap and irritate tender skin. Just make sure the gloves are long enough to prevent water and chemicals from splashing inside.

When it comes to gardening, dehydrating dirt isn't the only threat from which your hands need protection. Garden tools can be the source of blisters and calluses. Mower blades, edgers, trimmers, and other power equipment can inflict nasty cuts. More dangerous still, pesticides, herbicides, and chemical fertilizers are carcinogens, neurotoxins, and endocrine disruptors, which may cause long-term health problems. While it is best to use organic methods to control weeds and garden pests, if you must use these poisons, you'll get the most protection from gloves made of heavy canvas, cowhide, or suede. Make it a habit to inspect them before each use, and throw away or repair any with splits, tears, or holes.

Helping Hands

Although prevention is always easier than repairing damage already done, there are times when our hands need a bit of extra pampering. Despite our best efforts, dryness, irritation, and other common problems can periodically plague our hands. This section details some natural ways to give troubled hands the care they deserve.

Age Spots

Perhaps because our hands are exposed to the sun more than any other part of our body, they seem to be the first area to show the signs of aging. Unfortunately, the cumulative effect of naked, sunbaked hands is unattractive pools of dark pigment, known as age spots. While it's a good idea to apply a bit of zinc oxide–based sunblock to the back of the hands before heading outdoors, it's something we rarely think of doing until it's too late.

If age spots plague your hands, don't head to your drugstore for a jar of chemical-filled vanishing or bleaching creams. Gradually fade age spots naturally with undiluted lemon juice. Or try juicing some strawberries, pineapple, or papaya. Along with fading the unsightly spots, these alpha hydroxy–rich fruits will soften the skin. Simply dab the juice on the age spots once or twice a day with a cotton ball. Store the leftover juice in the refrigerator.

Contact Dermatitis

Often triggered by the ingredients in cosmetics, perfumes, personal care products, and household cleansers, contact dermatitis is an allergic reaction that can produce inflammation, flaking, thickening, weeping, color changes, and itching. Whatever the irritant, repeated contact with the offending substance can cause the dermatitis to worsen and spread. It is important to identify the source of irritation, if possible. If you have recently begun using a new product, it may be a simple task to pinpoint and eliminate the irritant. Unfortunately, it isn't always that easy. If you can't readily target the source of your dermatitis, a trip to a qualified dermatologist may be called for.

Once you have identified the culprit, check product labels and stop using any product containing the offending ingredient. In the meantime, several herbal remedies can alleviate some of the discomfort and speed healing when applied topically. Aloe vera gel can stem the inflammation that often accompanies contact dermatitis, say researchers at the Universidad Nacional Autonoma de Mexico in Tlalnepantla. According to the study, the gooey gel reduces swelling by inhibiting cyclooxygenase activity.[13] Cyclooxygenase is a naturally occurring enzyme that creates prostaglandins, hormonelike substances that modulate inflammation. Other herbs known for their anti-inflammatory properties include calendula and witch hazel. To relieve itching, try dabbing the affected area with a cotton ball soaked in chamomile tea.

Excessive Dryness

It doesn't take much to sap moisture from hardworking hands. A simple change in the weather can dehydrate your hands if you are prone to dry skin. Conventional cosmetic companies try to convince dry-skin sufferers that they need deep conditioning or advanced healing therapy found only in the company's product. However, despite the hype, these "heavy-duty" hand treatments are nothing more than a thick hand cream. For an intensive two-part treatment, gently exfoliate dry, flaky skin away with a bit of cornmeal. Once you've gotten rid of the dead skin cells, mix up one of the hand masks offered in the formula section later in the chapter. Slather it generously on your hands, don a pair of white cotton gloves, and leave it on for several hours or overnight to give the ingredients a chance to penetrate the skin. After washing away the residue, massage your hands with a natural moisturizer or hand lotion for incredibly smooth, soft skin.

Scars

Occasionally we suffer from a minor cut or burn that can, if untreated, leave a scar. To prevent or limit the amount of scarring produced as the injured tissue heals itself, massage some liquid vitamin E or lavender essential oil into the cut or burn.

Another remedy for burns that many cooks keep handy is aloe vera. Several studies have documented that the gel from this cactuslike succulent speeds healing by boosting circulation, increasing the formation of collagen, and reducing inflammation. Aloe vera can also ease the pain associated with a burn, thanks to its high content of salicylic acid, the main constituent in aspirin. Other studies have shown that aloe also influences the formation of fibrous tissue, an important quality when it comes to preventing scars. To treat a burn with aloe, gently smooth the pure gel over the injured area several times a day. If you are fortunate enough to have an aloe vera plant nearby, simply break off the tip of one of the outer leaves, peel back the skin, and rub the cool, gooey inner substance over the burn.

Sweaty Palms

At some time in our lives, we've all experienced that embarrassing wetness that springs forth from the palms of our hands. Sweaty palms are often a nervous reaction to uncomfortable situations such as job interviews or giving a speech. To dry up moist hands, try sprinkling cornstarch or arrowroot on the palms of your hands. If you are frequently plagued by sweaty palms, fill a small atomizer or spray bottle with witch hazel, and spritz your hands several times a day. Witch hazel is a natural astringent that can reduce the flow of moisture.

Nail Know-How

The last few decades have seen fingernails rise to such prominence in the world of beauty that an entire industry has grown up around them. Millions of women spend countless hours and even more money in nail salons, trying to achieve what they can't gain on their own—ten perfectly manicured nails. Yet, our nails are more than just a fashion accessory. They are a reflection of our health and well-being.

Your fingernails also make a powerful statement about how you see yourself. Dirty nails sporting chipped polish and ragged cuticles paint a picture of slovenliness. Healthy, meticulously groomed nails tell the world that you care about yourself down to the last detail.

Our nails are our fingertips' protective armor, guarding them against injury and infection. Made up of layers of a hard, fibrous protein called keratin, the nail rests on a fleshy pad of skin, known as the nail bed. At the base of the nail bed is the matrix, from which all new nail growth springs. The cuticle, a thin strip of flexible skin, protects the matrix from dirt and bacteria, which could result in an infection.

Nails grow approximately 1/500 to 1/20 of an inch a week—one reason it seems to take an eternity to achieve long nails. In fact, it can take from seven to nine months to grow a new nail from the cuticle to the tip of the finger.

The condition of your nails is an excellent indicator of inner health. The nails can reflect bad habits, such as smoking, as well as nutritional deficiencies. For example, hangnails can indicate a deficiency in protein, folic acid, or vitamin C. White spots can point to a need for more vitamin B_6 or zinc. And peeling nails can mean low levels of vitamins A and C or calcium.[14]

Troubled nails can also signal an underlying medical problem. Brittle nails can indicate a potential thyroid problem, impaired kidney function, or circulatory problems. Yellow nails can be a sign of liver or respiratory disorders or diabetes.[15] If the appearance of your nails changes suddenly for no apparent reason, check with your doctor.

Although poor health and diet can negatively impact our fingernails, most of the problems our nails experience are self-inflicted. How often do you find yourself using your nails as a tool to open a pop-top can or to scrape away the remains of a sticker or label? Or plunge your hands into a sink of hot soapy water? Even the cosmetics designed to help nails look their best can cause harm to both your nails and your health.

Toxic Tints

When it comes to making your nails dazzle, you can pick your poison, as the saying goes. Red, pink, blue—every color in the rainbow and then some. Even though nails can make a strong fashion statement, nail products are among the most toxic cosmetics on the market. Since our nails are extremely porous, capable of absorbing twenty to twenty-five times their weight in water, they can also absorb the chemicals used in nail polishes, removers, and cuticle creams.

Although it's fun to paint our nails different colors (after all, how often can you really change something on a whim?), the consequences are nothing to laugh at. Along with synthetic colors, conventional nail polish contains various resins, plasticizers, and preservatives. According to the FDA, complaints stemming from nail polish use include irritation and splitting of the nail, discolored nails, nails permanently stained black, and nausea. Allergic reactions are also common and can affect not only the nails but also your skin, eyelids, and neck. But the health effects of the chemicals in nail products can go far beyond a simple case of discoloration or allergic reaction. Let's take a look at what's really in that bottle of shell pink or ruby red polish.

One of the most dangerous components in nail polish is toluene. Toluene is used primarily as a solvent and can comprise 50 percent of the ingredients in some brands of polish. Derived from petroleum crude, toluene affects the central nervous system. Long-term exposure to low levels can cause fatigue, confusion, memory loss, tingling in the fingers and toes, nausea, and loss of appetite, as well as skin irritation and respiratory problems. But can a quick paint job really expose you to unsafe levels of this neurotoxin? Yes, say experts at the U.S. Department of Health and Human Services Agency for Toxic Substances and Disease Registry, who note that high exposure can occur from the home use of nail polish.[16] The Environmental Protection Agency's Office of Pollution Prevention and Toxics concurs, warning that breathing large amounts of toluene for short periods can adversely affect the kidneys, the liver, and the heart.[17]

Currently toluene is regulated under California's Proposition 65 as a developmental toxin. Studies of rats and mice exposed to toluene show that this chemical can cause spontaneous abortion and delay skeletal development in fetuses. A study in Japan, where toluene is considered an abused substance, found that inhalation caused neurobehavorial effects.[18] In addition, several studies have found that women exposed occupationally were five times more likely to experience spontaneous abortion than unexposed women.[19] Despite the evidence, the Cosmetic Ingredient Review Panel (CIR), an industry-run organization charged with investigating the safety of cosmetics, has deemed toluene safe as currently used.

Formaldehyde is another chemical with a long history of use in nail polish. Employed mainly as an inexpensive preservative and antibacterial, it is one of the volatile organic compounds that has been classified as a human carcinogen. Although formaldehyde is a common addition in nail polish and hardeners, researchers from the National Cancer Institute recommended further study as far back as 1983 since this highly reactive chemical can cause

DNA damage and may combine with other chemicals to produce mutagenic effects.[20]

Formaldehyde exposure can result in severe asthmatic reactions, skin rashes, and hives. According to a 1997 consumer update released by the Consumer Product Safety Commission, exposure to airborne formaldehyde at levels above 0.1 part per million can also cause watery or burning eyes, nausea, coughing, tightness in the chest, and wheezing.[21] Moreover, you needn't breathe the vapors to become exposed. Formaldehyde can be absorbed into the skin when the chemical is in its liquid state. Because formaldehyde poses such a health risk, this chemical is banned in Japan and Sweden.[22]

Combining the best of both worlds, toluene-sulfonamide/formaldehyde resin is a plasticizer that improves the adhesion and gloss of nail polish. It is also used as a nail hardener in strengthening formulas. A strong sensitizer in its liquid state, it can cause a reaction upon skin contact. Oddly enough, allergic reactions to this chemical rarely show up at the point of contact. Instead of appearing on the hands and nails, reactions target the eyelids, the sides of the neck, and areas around the mouth.

Fortunately, a number of nail polish manufacturers have bowed to consumer concern by removing toluene and formaldehyde from their products. But there is another, more potentially damaging, chemical found in nail polish. Dibutyl phthalate, or DBP, is a developmental toxin that affects the testes in men. Although the CIR believes DBP is safe when applied topically, recent studies have found this plasticizer to be an estrogenic chemical that may accelerate sexual development. A study of young Puerto Rican girls found that long-term exposure to DBP resulted in premature breast development.[23] Other reproductive effects in women exposed to phthalates in the workplace include menstrual disorders, miscarriages, and premature births. Also, in numerous animal studies, DBP has been found to be responsible for fetal deformities such as a cleft palate or undescended testicles.

All phthalates are easily absorbed by the skin and tend to accumulate in the body's fatty tissue, although some of this accumulation is broken down and excreted by the body. A recent study by researchers at the Centers for Disease Control (CDC) National Center for Environmental Health found that women in their childbearing years had particularly high urinary levels of DBP and strongly urged that the health risks be reassessed.[24]

If your fingertips simply must sport color, a new technology may be just what you are looking for. Nontoxic water-based polishes offer color without many of the hazardous solvents and resins found in conventional products. Free from synthetic resins, these products discourage chipping, allow the nail to breathe, and don't require a polish remover to take them off. When you are ready to remove your polish, you simply peel the color from your nails. On the downside, nontoxic polishes are still a developing industry, so quality may be an issue. While some brands rival conventional polishes for their ease of application and durability, others don't yet offer the high gloss or smooth surface that most women expect from their polish. The best advice is to try several brands until you find one you like.

Macabre Manicure

Now that you're ready to toss out all those bottles of nail polish, what about removing the polish already on your fingernails? Although different formulations contain different ingredients, one constant in all conventional nail polish removers is acetone. Frequent use of an acetone-based nail polish remover can dry out nails and may cause brittleness, peeling, and splitting. Short-term exposure to this strong solvent may also cause a skin rash.

You can detect the presence of acetone by its distinctive odor. The powerful acrid smell should be a warning. When inhaled, acetone makes its way into the blood, where it is carried to all of the other organs. While small amounts are broken down by the liver, exposure to moderate-to-high levels can cause nose, throat, lung, and eye irritation, headaches, light-headedness, confusion, increased pulse rate, nausea, vomiting, unconsciousness, and possibly coma. Animal studies show that long-term exposure not only damages the kidneys, liver, and nervous system but also increases the occurrence of birth defects.

And what about those creams that claim to whisk away ragged cuticles? No matter how rich and creamy conventional cuticle removers may seem, they contain a mix of synthetic moisturizers and caustic ingredients, such as lye or potassium hydroxide, to soften and remove cuticles. Potassium hydroxide is extremely corrosive and may cause contact dermatitis and burning. In fact, products with concentrations of 5 percent or more can actually destroy fingernails.[25] A much safer way to control creeping cuticles is to gently push them back with a towel after your bath or shower and moisturize with a bit of vitamin E or olive oil.

Fakin' It

You've seen them. You may even have them. Long, perfectly manicured sculptured nails. In 1999 alone, American women spent more than $4 billion on artificial nails, making it the most requested salon service.[26] Yet, the lengths to which some women will go to have beautiful nails can expose them to some heavy-duty toxins and leave the door open to serious infection and nail damage.

When acrylic nails first burst upon the scene in the 1970s, they were made from methyl methacrylate (MMA). The use of MMA to create "porcelain nails" provided manicurists with a strong, long-lasting way to extend short nails and cover up damaged or discolored nails. But as the popularity of acrylic nails increased, so did the problems. Users reported skin allergies, numbness in the fingers, and permanent nail deformities. Worse yet, MMA was found to be potentially carcinogenic, and long-term use could cause permanent damage to the respiratory tract and nervous system. By the end of the '70s, the FDA had received so many complaints related to the use of MMA, the agency banned its use in nail products, stating that the chemical was "a poisonous and deleterious substance."

Since consumer demand for acrylic nails was so high, the industry quickly found substitutes for MMA. The most widely used substitute used today is ethyl methacrylate (EMA). While not a banned substance, EMA carries health risks similar to those associated with MMA. Short-term health effects include contact dermatitis and allergic reactions affecting the nose, throat, eyes, and mucous membranes. And having your nails done in a poorly ventilated space can cause dizziness and light-headedness. Your nail technician may be at even greater risk. According to a study by the CDC, occupational exposure to EMA can cause asthma.[27] Several other studies have linked long-term EMA use to birth defects, neurological damage, and cancer in animals.

Another dubious substance associated with acrylic nails is methyl ethyl ketone (MEK). Designated by the Occupational Safety and Health Administration as a hazardous substance, MEK is a solvent used to make vinyl adhesives, resins, and acrylics. It is also present in some nail polishes. Breathing MEK for even a few minutes can irritate the eyes, nose, and throat and may cause headaches, dizziness, nausea, and numbness in the fingers and toes. Extreme exposure may lead to personality changes, sleep disturbances, reduced coordination, and unconsciousness. A strong irritant, MEK can also be absorbed by the skin, where, according to the Material Safety Data Sheet, it may have systemic effects.[28] Repeated exposure can also cause drying and cracking of the skin. According to the New Jersey Department of Health and Senior Services Right to Know Program, there is limited evidence that MEK causes birth defects in animals and should be treated as a possible teratogen in humans.[29]

Even without these chemical risks, sculptured acrylic nails have never been a wholesome option. Nails need to "breathe" in order to be healthy. When nails are covered with a plastic resin, the normal oxygen exchange needed to keep them strong is prevented. Without the ability to breathe, your nails become weak, thin, and yellow.

Infection is also a common problem. A study by the University of Michigan concluded that health care workers wearing artificial fingernails harbored significantly more harmful bacteria and yeasts than their unadorned counterparts.[30] Based on this study, some hospitals have banned the use of artificial nails, especially in surgical departments. Because artificial nails are such a welcoming haven for these biological critters, bacterial and yeast infections occur frequently. If untreated, these infections can cause the nail to become spongy or mushy and may result in the loss of the nail.

Another common problem with sculptured nails is fungal infections. Moisture can become trapped underneath the artificial nail, creating an inviting home for fungal growth. Most dermatologists recommend taking a one-month vacation from acrylic nails every three to six months to give them a chance to breathe and recover from the toll that artificial nails take on the real thing.

When it comes time to remove acrylic nails, you may think you're home free. Not so. Dislodging the sculptured nail from your own requires an extremely powerful solvent. Acetonitrile is the solvent of choice. Toxic when inhaled or absorbed through the skin, acetonitrile breaks down into cyanide when swallowed, making it particularly dangerous to children. In 1987, a sixteen-month-old California boy died of cyanide poisoning after swallowing a mouthful of acetonitrile.[31] He is not alone. In 1990, nearly twenty-nine hundred children, age four and under, were rushed to the emergency room because they consumed nail products.[32] Little wonder, since artificial nail removers contain at least 98 percent acetonitrile.

Although the FDA acknowledges the dangers of products containing this lethal solvent, the agency is powerless to take action. Unlike household cleaners, which are allowed to contain concentrations of cyanide no greater than

25 parts per million, artificial nail removers are considered cosmetics and can legally contain 4,000 to 80,000 parts per million of this cyanide equivalent.[33] Since acetonitrile-based nail removers are carried in most beauty supply stores, the danger is widespread; parents need to read the label and take special precautions to keep the product away from children.

Acetonitrile also poses a danger for adults. This irritant can affect the eyes, nose, throat, skin, and lungs, and repeated exposure may cause an enlarged thyroid. The New Jersey Department of Health and Senior Services also notes that chronic exposure can cause reproductive damage and warns that acetonitrile should be handled with extreme caution.[34]

If sculptured nails don't seem worth the health risks but you still love the look of long, lovely nails, the nail industry has an alternative that, on the surface, seems like a safer option. But don't be fooled. The preformed, press-on plastic nails available at your local drugstore aren't much better than expensive acrylics. The culprits aren't the nails themselves but the glues used to attach them. Speaking at the 1997 meeting of the American Academy of Dermatology, Zoe Draelos, M.D., clinical professor in the Department of Dermatology at the Bowman Gray School of Medicine, warned: "Stronger nail adhesives are used to provide better adhesion but can cause the nail plate to separate from the nail bed. In addition, traumatic removal of artificial nails may result in the nail plate splitting into layers."[35]

One of the most common adhesives used to attach plastic nails is cyanoacrylate, the same chemical used in superglue. A study by the University of Arkansas found that cyanoacrylate adhesives were directly linked to nail discoloration and malformation. The researchers also found that people sensitive to these glues suffered from allergic contact dermatitis and eczema of the fingertips. Adhesive-related eczema was also found in other areas of the body, probably due to contact with the nails.[36] Some users have also complained of dizziness, headaches, and shortness of breath when using cyanoacrylate glue.

While it's tough to have fire-engine red talons decorated with glitter or gold without the use of these toxic tools, you can have beautiful, well-groomed nails naturally.

Finger Food

Having healthy nails free from hangnails, brittleness, cracks, ridges, white spots, or peeling edges depends on a good diet. The proper diet not only supports good circulation and healthy nail growth but also can help keep problems at bay.

Which nutrients are vital to growing a set of healthy nails? Topping the list is biotin, one of the B vitamins. Biotin not only helps the body utilize the other B vitamins but also promotes the growth of healthy cells and nerve tissue and has a direct impact on the health of your cuticles. A deficiency can cause scaling of the cuticles, brittleness, and nail ridges. Present in brewer's yeast, milk, soybeans, whole grains, poultry, and seafood, biotin also helps metabolize protein.

A good source of protein is also vital to healthy nails. The best sources include lean meat, poultry, fish, beans, whole grains, nuts, and seeds. Once consumed, protein is broken down into the amino acids needed to build the nails themselves.

Calcium is another important nail nutrient. We all know calcium's reputation for promoting strong bones and teeth, but this mineral also prevents brittle nails. Good sources include salmon, dairy foods, and dark green leafy vegetables.

In addition, healthy nails need lubrication to keep them glossy and supple. The best sources of this lubrication are essential fatty acids (EFAs). Unlike many other dietary fats, EFAs are essential to good health and promote the normal growth of blood vessels and nerves, two critical factors in proper nail growth and function. Although you can supplement your diet with EFA-rich primrose oil, adding flaxseed or canola oil and cold freshwater fish such as salmon to your diet can be a delicious way to achieve glowing nails.

Another important nutrient on the nail hit parade is silica. A component of many popular nail supplements, silica gives nails their strength and stability. Since this mineral is easily lost in food processing, you can either use one of the supplements on the market or look for unprocessed wheat, alfalfa, avocados, strawberries, and dark leafy greens. A silica-rich herb, such as horsetail or oat straw, can also be brewed as a tea and sipped throughout the day. Other nail-friendly nutrients include vitamins A, C, and E; folic acid; zinc; and a good vitamin B complex.

Although no single nutrient is a magic bullet for beautiful nails, there is one supplement that may hold promise for boosting your nail's health and appearance. Methylsulfonylmethane, commonly known as MSM, is an organic sulfur compound naturally present in the human body. Reputed as the "beauty mineral," sulfur is essential for strong nails. The key component in sulfur is cystine, the amino acid responsible for giving keratin its strength. Although MSM is in many foods, because our diets contain such a large proportion of highly processed foods, it's not uncommon for people to be deficient in MSM. Anecdotal evidence indicates that supplementing the diet with 2,000 milligrams a day may help restore strength and flexibility to nails.[37]

Water is another important part of a nail-healthy diet. Drinking plenty of water boosts the nails' natural moisture, keeping them from becoming brittle. Water is fundamental as well in transporting all of the essential nutrients cited here to our nails. Drinking at least eight 8-ounce glasses of water a day helps ensure that your nails are getting the moisture they need.

Natural Nail Tips

Although consuming water is critical to maintaining healthy nails, exposing our nails to a sink full of hot water has the opposite effect. Since our nails are so porous, repeated exposure can cause the keratin fibers to swell and split apart. When waterlogged nails dry, they contract and become dehydrated. The result can be soft, brittle nails that break at the drop of a hat. The solution? Always wear rubber or latex gloves when exposing your nails to water, particularly hot water containing household cleaners.

Treating your nails with kindness can go a long way toward keeping them healthy and attractive. A few minutes of daily pampering will reap more benefits than hours spent at the nail salon. To keep unruly cuticles in line, gently push them back every time you wash your hands or apply hand cream. It's a habit that will pay off when you do your weekly manicure. Keeping your nails and cuticles moisturized is another habit that is worth developing and takes only seconds. Before bed, simply massage a bit of liquid vitamin E into your nails. Your nails will glow with health!

Here are a few more tips to help you develop beautiful nails:

- **Don't** try to clean dirt from under the nails with a sharp object. You can injure the delicate nail bed and invite a nasty infection. Use a nail brush instead.
- **Don't** use a seesaw motion when you file your nails. The back-and-forth motion of the file can cause nails to split and develop ridges. File in one

direction only, from the outer edge to the center, using long, smooth strokes.

- **Don't** pull off a torn or split nail. Doing so can damage the surrounding nail and cause peeling. Snip off the offending damage with nail scissors or a clipper, and then file the nail smooth.
- **Don't** cut your cuticles—ever! Vigorous cutting can lead to inflammation, hangnails, and ragged, bleeding cuticles that can become infected.
- **Don't** allow your nails to get too long. A study by the University of Texas found that longer nails reduce the speed of finger manipulation, range of motion, and grip strength. For optimal finger function, the researchers suggest that fingernails be kept at 0.5 centimeter, or slightly less than one-half inch, past the tip of the finger.[38]

The Perfect Ten

A good weekly manicure isn't an indulgence; it's a necessity required to eliminate snags and rough edges, nourish the cuticles, and keep your nails looking their best. Here are six easy steps to beautifully manicured nails:

1. **File your nails into an attractive shape.** Using a nonmetallic file or emery board, file each nail from corner to center, tilting the file under the nail slightly to reduce frayed edges.
2. **Clean your nails.** Using a soft natural-bristle nail brush, gently scrub your nails with soap and water. Clean the tops of the nails and the cuticles, and then move to the underside of the nail, making sure you remove any accumulated dirt.
3. **Soak your nails.** Choose from the formulas located at the end of this chapter to remove any traces of dirt and debris from your nails.
4. **Apply a cuticle cream.** This will moisturize and soften the cuticles. After a few minutes, gently push back the cuticles, using a soft damp towel.
5. **Condition your hands.** Massage a generous helping of hand cream into your hands until all traces have been absorbed.
6. **Add some shine with a chamois buffer.** These are available from most beauty supply stores. Dab a bit of olive oil or buffing cream onto the nail, and buff vigorously in one direction. Buffing stimulates circulation, giving your nails a soft, healthy sheen.

Hell on Heels

As much as we abuse our hands and nails, our feet often bear the brunt of total neglect. Rough heels, corns, and calluses can make our feet look less than alluring. And, according to the American Podiatric Medical Association, 75 percent of Americans complain of foot pain or infection some time in their lives.[39] The encouraging news is that much of the suffering our tired tootsies endure can be prevented with proper care.

Since the most common cause of foot pain is our footwear, the path to healthy feet begins at the shoe store. Topping the list of bad choices is high heels. A recent pilot study by the British College of Naturopathy and Osteopathy found that women who wear heels higher than two inches have a greater risk of developing hammertoes, corns, and calluses.[40] Another problem is that high heels shift the weight of the body onto the ball of the foot. Over time, this type of shoe may cause enough change in the feet to impair their proper function.

The key to healthy footwear is proper fit. The APMA recommends checking your shoe size each time you buy shoes and doing your buying at the end of the day, when feet are the most swollen. If you must wear elevated heels, opt for a pump under two inches, with a broad base to stabilize your weight, and avoid pointy shoes that force you to scrunch five toes into a space designed for four.

Foot Fixes

Neglect and abuse can result in a variety of painful, yet common, foot ailments. One of the most common is blisters, a condition caused by friction on the skin. You can easily prevent blisters by wearing two layers of socks, but if you do find yourself afflicted, make a small hole at the edge of the blister with a sterilized needle, and then gently push the fluid out while keeping the skin intact. Clean the area thoroughly, and spray it with tea tree oil before bandaging.

Corns and calluses can also cause foot misery. Normally, our feet absorb about five hundred pounds of pressure with each step we take. When we subject them to excessive pressure such as jogging, thick growths, known as corns and calluses, may appear. Corns usually occur over joints, such as the toes, while calluses occur on the bottom of the foot. Fortunately, a good exfoliant will help relieve tough calluses. To treat corns at home, massage castor oil into the area or soak your feet in a solution of warm water and nondistilled apple cider vinegar daily until the problem disappears. Never cut a corn or callus, and avoid medicated pads and paints that promise to remove the problem. These remedies contain salicylic acid and can burn the healthy tissue surrounding the affected area.

A more serious problem is bunions, deformities that cause the first long bone in the foot to turn inward and the big toe to turn outward. Although often hereditary, bunions are aggravated by tight shoes and high heels. A warm footbath may help relieve the pain and swelling, but severe cases may require surgery. Since bunions can also lead to ingrown toenails, corns, and hammertoes (a condition that permanently bends the smaller toes into a claw shape), properly fitting shoes with a wide toe box are essential.

Fungal First Aid

Athlete's foot is probably the most common infection that afflicts feet. Despite its name, athlete's foot isn't just the curse of jocks. It can strike anyone as long as the conditions are right—warm, moist environments such as poorly ventilated shoes and damp sweaty socks.

While athlete's foot isn't life threatening, it can be painful. Symptoms include inflammation, burning, itching, scaly or cracked skin, and blisters. If you are prone to the disease, make sure you keep your feet clean and dry. Adding zinc-rich foods, such as nuts and seeds, to your diet can also inhibit the fungus and help stimulate your immune system.

If you are past the point of prevention, don't automatically reach for a mainstream remedy. Over-the-counter athlete's foot remedies may contain miconazole, an antifungal that can cause irritation, burning, and itching—the very symptoms you are trying to relieve![41] Another popular ingredient is benzethonium chloride, a detergent included for its antiseptic properties. In 1992, the FDA issued a warning that this chemical has not been shown to be safe and effective in over-the-counter remedies.[42] For an effective nontoxic approach, try a topical application of colloidal silver. A natural antibiotic and disinfectant, colloidal silver destroys fungi and bacteria while it promotes healing.

Another alternative to chemical treatments is the powerful antifungal herb tea tree oil. Use it straight, applying it to the affected area, or soak your feet in a small tub of warm water to which twenty drops of tea tree oil have been added. Garlic is also a potent antifungal, rivaling nonprescription foot powders for effectiveness. Simply rub a clove of crushed garlic between your toes, and dust your shoes and socks with garlic powder.

Unfortunately, fungal infections aren't limited to the crevices between the toes. Discolored, brittle, or raised toenails can be a sign of a toenail infection. These unsightly infections are caused by parasitic fungi, yeasts, or molds. The affected nail appears yellow-brownish-gray and can have a worm-eaten look. Although this type of infection is painless, if left untreated, it can eventually destroy the nail.

Tackle stubborn nail fungi with a liquid garlic extract, and as an extra measure, add an aged garlic supplement to your diet. A tea tree oil footbath or a soak in an herbal infusion of pau d'arco and goldenseal will also help kill the fungi. To make a pau d'arco footbath, wrap 6 tablespoons of the herb in cheesecloth. Secure the packet, and cover it with a gallon of boiling water. Let it steep for 20 minutes before adding 20 drops of goldenseal essential oil. Soak your feet in this solution for 15 minutes twice a day.

Toe Woes

Although an ingrown toenail may not sound like a big deal, it can literally keep you off your feet. Often caused by improper cutting or by wearing shoes and socks that are too tight, an ingrown toenail is inflamed, red, and very tender. For a minor ingrown toenail, soak your foot daily to keep the flesh around the nail soft and pliable. To prevent infection, apply a topical antibiotic such as liquid garlic. Whatever you do, don't poke at the nail or try to pry it away from the skin. If treated improperly, an ingrown toenail may require attention from your health care provider or perhaps even minor surgery.

Smooth Steppin'

Dry, scaly skin can make feet uncomfortable and unattractive. What's more, chronic dry skin can lead to cracks and fissures—an open invitation to bacteria and infection. Yet, just a few minutes of daily pampering with a good-quality moisturizer can prevent dryness and leave your feet soft and smooth. But be warned that moisturizers and foot creams contain the same synthetic petrochemicals and preservatives that are in hand creams and lotions.

For a super softening treatment, try this bedtime strategy: Soak your feet in warm water until the skin softens. Adding a handful of oatmeal wrapped in cheesecloth enhances the softening process. Gently rub problem areas with a scrub or a wet pumice stone to remove the dead skin. If you have excessively dry feet, it may take more than one soaking to remove all the dead skin. Follow up with a thick coating of moisturizer and, using the same principle as the overnight hand treatment, cover with thick white cotton socks. By morning, the moisturizer will have been absorbed and your feet will be sleek and silky.

The Pampering Pedicure

You don't have to visit a salon to achieve beautiful feet. In fact, professional procedures such as cutting the nails or cuticles can break the skin and may put you at risk of contracting a fungal or bacterial infection.[43] For a natural do-it-yourself pedicure, follow these simple steps:

1. **Soak your feet.** Use warm water mixed with a few drops of lavender essential oil. Gently rub your feet with a pumice stone to remove dead skin.
2. **Moisturize with a natural cream or lotion.** Gently massage your feet until all of the moisturizer has been absorbed.
3. **Trim toenails.** With a toenail clipper, cut the nails straight across to prevent ingrown nails. Smooth rough edges with an emery board.
4. **Apply a cuticle cream.** After a few minutes, gently push the cuticles back with a damp towel.
5. **Perk up your toenails.** Apply a coat of water-based nail polish, or buff them to a low sheen for a natural look.

By making smart choices and giving your feet the regular care they deserve, you will not only keep your feet beautiful but also help ensure a healthy, pain-free foundation for life. Table 6.1 includes herbal remedies for both foot and hand problems.

Table 6.1 🍃 Herbal Remedies for Hand and Foot Problems

Exposure to the elements, harsh chemicals, and simple neglect can add up to problems when it comes to hands and feet. Instead of turning to chemically packed remedies, try natural products containing these age-old herbal helpers.

If You Have . . .	Useful Herbs	Comments and Cautions
athlete's foot	garlic, goldenseal, pau d'arco, tea tree oil	Keep the area between the toes dry between treatments.
blisters	lavender, tea tree oil	
chapped skin	cucumber, geranium, marshmallow, rose, slippery elm	
dry nails	aloe vera, geranium, rose	
dry skin	aloe vera, calendula, cucumber, rose, slippery elm	
foot odor	chamomile, sage	
fungal infections	garlic, goldenseal, pau d'arco, tea tree oil, thyme	
peeling nails	wheat germ oil	
soft nails	horsetail, oat straw	
tired feet	clove, eucalyptus, peppermint	
warts	aloe vera, black walnut, clove, goldenseal, pau d'arco, wintergreen	Apply 3 times daily for several weeks.

Homemade Hand and Foot Care

Well-nourished and healthy hands, feet, and nails can rarely be had from the products you find at the cosmetics counter. Although these products may offer short-term solutions, for a lifetime of beautiful hands and feet, adopt a regular routine using any of the formulas in this section.

Hand Care

Daily care can keep hands from becoming rough and dry. Moisturize several times a day, particularly after exposing hands to water. For hands that work hard, try a weekly treatment using one of the exfoliators or masks designed to keep hands soft and supple.

Rich Rose Hand Cream   YIELD: 8 ounces
Slather on this fragrant antioxidant-rich cream to keep hands petal soft.

¼ cup rose petals
1 tablespoon rose hips
½ cup hot, not boiling, distilled water
1 tablespoon beeswax, grated
1 tablespoon cocoa butter
½ cup almond oil
1 teaspoon liquid vitamin E
7 drops rose essential oil

Place the petals and rose hips in a glass bowl and crush gently with the back of a wooden spoon. Cover with hot water and allow to steep overnight. Strain the liquid into a glass container and set aside. Discard the petals and rose hips.

In a small double boiler over medium heat, melt the beeswax and cocoa butter, stirring constantly. Add the almond oil, and whisk until thoroughly mixed. Remove from heat and cool slightly. Mix in the reserved rose liquid, the vitamin E, and the rose essential oil and stir gently until well blended, or use a blender to emulsify the mixture. Cool completely and pour into a sterilized glass jar with a tight-fitting lid.

Lavender Hand Lotion   YIELD: 8 ounces
Luscious lavender combines with healing calendula to soothe and soften dry skin. Keep a jar near the kitchen sink to banish dishpan hands.

½ cup aloe vera gel
1 tablespoon dried lavender flowers
1 tablespoon dried calendula flowers
¼ cup glycerin
¼ cup wheat germ oil
½ teaspoon beeswax, grated

    1 teaspoon liquid vitamin E
    5 drops lavender essential oil

Combine the aloe, lavender, calendula, glycerin, wheat germ oil, and beeswax in a small pan. Heat over a low flame, stirring gently, until the beeswax has melted completely. Strain, discarding the flowers. Cool and add the vitamin E and essential oil. Mix well before pouring into a clean jar with a tight-fitting lid.

Oatmeal Exfoliator

YIELD: 1 application

Exfoliators are great for removing dead skin cells, improving circulation, and moisturizing dehydrated skin. These treatments needn't be reserved for your face: use this once-a-week treatment to banish dry, rough hands.

    ½ cup oatmeal
    ¼ cup cornmeal
    ¼ cup honey

Mix the ingredients in a small glass bowl. Generously massage the mixture into hands, paying special attention to dry spots. Rinse with tepid water and follow with a good moisturizer.

Honey Hand Mask

YIELD: 1 application

Overexposure to weather, water, and harsh chemicals can leave hands in sad shape. For excessive dryness, try this heavy-duty overnight moisturizing treatment.

    ½ teaspoon avocado oil
    ½ teaspoon wheat germ oil
    ½ teaspoon jojoba oil
    ½ teaspoon liquid vitamin E
    2 tablespoons plain yogurt
    1 egg yolk

Combine the ingredients in a small glass bowl and whisk to blend. Store in the refrigerator until ready to use. Before bed, slather generously onto hands, and cover with a pair of white cotton gloves. The next morning, wash hands well with a nondrying, glycerin-based soap.

A Little Night Magic
YIELD: 1 application

Sometimes, just blending a couple of simple ingredients can give spectacular results.

> 1 teaspoon olive oil
> 1 teaspoon honey

Mix the oil and honey together in a small glass bowl. Massage into your hands just before bed and don a pair of white cotton gloves. The next morning, wash hands well with a nondrying, glycerin-based soap.

Avocado Butter Hand Mask
YIELD: 1 application

If an overnight hand mask isn't practical, try this 20-minute emollient-rich mask before your next manicure.

> ½ ripe avocado
> 1 teaspoon avocado oil
> ½ teaspoon liquid vitamin E

Place the ingredients in a food processor and puree. Massage into hands, and then slip them into a pair of disposable plastic gloves. Relax for 20 minutes before rinsing hands well in tepid water. Pat dry and manicure. (Tip: Instead of tossing the plastic gloves, rinse and dry thoroughly. Store them with your manicure supplies, and they will be ready for reuse.)

Lemon Lightener
YIELD: 4 ounces

Used daily, this lemony hand cream will help fade discolorations, freckles, and age spots.

> ½ teaspoon prepared horseradish
> 1 tablespoon aloe vera gel
> 1 teaspoon fresh lemon juice
> 1 tablespoon beeswax, grated
> 1 tablespoon glycerin
> 1 teaspoon liquid vitamin E
> 3 drops lemon essential oil

Mix the horseradish, aloe, and lemon juice in a small glass bowl and set aside. In a small saucepan over a low flame, heat the beeswax and glycerin until the beeswax has melted. Cool and combine with the reserved horseradish mixture, blending well. Once the mixture has cooled completely, add the vitamin E and essential oil, mixing thoroughly. Pour into a clean glass jar with a tight-fitting lid. To use, massage into discolored areas.

Ageless Hands Alpha Hydroxy Cream   YIELD: 4 ounces
Turn back the clock with this exfoliating hand lotion designed to fade unsightly age spots. This cream must be refrigerated to prevent spoilage.

¼ cup strawberries
¼ cup papaya, peeled and cubed
1 to 2 tablespoons distilled water
1 tablespoon beeswax, grated
1 tablespoon cocoa butter
½ cup almond oil
1 teaspoon liquid vitamin E
10,000 international units vitamin A, crushed
500 milligrams vitamin C, crushed
5 drops rose geranium essential oil

Place the strawberries and papaya in a food processor with just enough water to process. Process until smooth, and set aside.

In a small saucepan, gently heat the beeswax, cocoa butter, and almond oil until the beeswax has melted completely. Remove from heat. In a glass bowl, thoroughly mix together the reserved fruit puree and beeswax mixture. Add the vitamins E, A, and C and essential oil, and mix again until well blended. Pour into a glass jar with a tight-fitting lid. Use as you would any other hand cream.

Nail Helpers

Some women spend a fortune to attain long, beautiful nails—money often wasted on toxic products that can result in damage. Opt instead for natural nails, using the toxic-free formulas featured here to pamper cuticles and encourage healthy new growth.

Cocoa Butter Cuticle Oil   YIELD: 2 ounces

Dry cuticles can become ragged and split, allowing dirt and germs to invade the matrix of the nail. Keep your cuticles soft and healthy with this chocolate-scented oil.

2 tablespoons jojoba oil
1 tablespoon wheat germ oil
1 tablespoon cocoa butter

Place the ingredients in a small saucepan. Heat gently until the cocoa butter has completely melted. Stir well and cool. Pour into a glass jar with a tight-fitting lid. To use, massage a small amount into the base of each nail, gently pushing back the cuticles.

Nail-Conditioning Oil   YIELD: ½ ounce

Regardless of how badly you've abused your nails, vitamin E can help restore them to health. To speed healing, massage this nutrient-rich oil into your nails each night before bed.

1½ teaspoons liquid vitamin E
1 teaspoon almond oil

Pour the vitamin E and almond oil into a small glass bottle. Cap and shake vigorously to mix. To use, massage a small amount into each nail, gently pushing back the cuticles.

Natural Nail Strengthener   YIELD: 4 ounces

Although chemically packed hardeners claim to be a quick fix for soft nails, this colorless henna-based formula will strengthen nails without chemicals. Remember, never use metal utensils when working with henna.

½ teaspoon horsetail
½ cup distilled water
1 teaspoon neutral henna

Wrap the horsetail in a square of cheesecloth and secure tightly with a rubber band. Pour the water into a glass measuring cup and add the horsetail packet. Boil the water in the microwave, 1 to 2 minutes on high.

Meanwhile, place the henna in a small glass bowl. Remove the horsetail packet from the boiling water and discard. Stirring constantly with a wooden or plastic spoon, add the water to the henna. Stir until the henna has dissolved. Cool, stirring occasionally, and pour into a clean glass jar with a tight-fitting lid. To use, shake the mixture to evenly distribute the henna. Apply to clean nails with a small paintbrush or cotton swab.

Tough-As-Nails Tea   YIELD: 1 serving
Drinking a cup or two of this internal nail treatment each day is a tasty way to achieve visibly stronger nails.

> 1 teaspoon dried horsetail, chopped
> 1 teaspoon dried oat straw, chopped
> ½ teaspoon dried lavender flowers
> 1 cup boiling distilled water
> Honey (optional)

Place the horsetail, oat straw, and lavender in a small tea ball, or wrap in a square of cheesecloth and secure with a rubber band. Set the tea ball or packet in the bottom of an attractive mug and add the boiling water. Steep for 5 to 7 minutes. Add honey if desired and enjoy!

Peeling-Nail Oil   YIELD: 1 application
Peeling nails can be a sign of a vitamin A, vitamin C, or calcium deficiency. They can also be the result of repeated exposure to the harsh solvents in conventional nail products. Check your diet, toss the toxic nail products, and try this treatment to discourage peeling and splitting.

> 1 teaspoon wheat germ oil
> ¼ teaspoon liquid vitamin E

Blend the oil and vitamin E well and massage into peeling nails daily.

Buffing Polish   YIELD: 1 application
Forget nail polish! Shorter nails can look terrific when buffed to a high shine. Buffing also stimulates circulation and promotes healthy nail growth.

> 1 tablespoon almond oil
> 1 teaspoon baking soda

Stir the oil and baking soda together until the baking soda has dissolved. To use, spread a small amount on each nail, and then buff to the desired shine with a chamois buffer.

Hardening Nail Soak   YIELD: 1 application
This silica-rich soak will help strengthen soft nails.

1 teaspoon horsetail
1 teaspoon oat straw
½ cup boiling distilled water

Place the horsetail and oat straw in a tea ball and set in the bottom of a small glass bowl. Cover with the boiling water and let steep for 10 minutes. Remove the tea ball and allow the liquid to cool until comfortably warm. Soak nails in the solution for 5 minutes. Dry hands with a soft towel, gently pushing back the cuticles.

Moisturizing Nail Soak   YIELD: 1 application
Dry, brittle nails? Try this honey and aloe vera soak before your next manicure to boost your nails' moisture content.

1 tablespoon honey
1 tablespoon aloe vera gel
½ cup boiling distilled water
1 teaspoon vitamin E
5 drops rose essential oil

Combine the honey, aloe, and boiling water in a small glass bowl, stirring to dissolve the honey and aloe. Cool until comfortably warm. Stir in the vitamin E and essential oil. Soak nails in the solution for 10 minutes. Dry hands with a soft towel, gently pushing back the cuticles.

Fungal-Fighting Nail Soak   YIELD: 1 application
Battling a nail fungus can be quite a challenge, one requiring strong antifungal herbs such as tea tree oil and thyme. To speed healing, let your nails breathe by keeping them polish-free, and use this antifungal nail soak every other day to send the fungus packing.

1 teaspoon fresh thyme, crushed
½ cup boiling distilled water
1 teaspoon tea tree oil

Place the thyme in a small bowl, pour the boiling water over the herb, and steep for 10 minutes. Cool until comfortably warm. Stir in the tea tree oil. Soak nails in the solution for 10 minutes. Dry hands and nails thoroughly with a clean, soft towel.

Foot Care

Feet are often the most forgotten part of the body. Neglect and abuse can team up to cause problems—from rough skin to painful conditions that require medical attention. Give your feet some long-overdue pampering with these simple formulas.

Almond Foot Smoother   YIELD: 1 application
Finely ground almonds combine with honey to smooth and moisturize dry, rough skin.

   ¼ cup finely ground almonds
   ¼ cup honey

Combine the almonds and honey in a small glass bowl, mixing well. Massage into feet, concentrating on particularly rough spots such as the heels.

Corny Foot Scrub   YIELD: 1 application
Cornmeal is a good, inexpensive exfoliant for softening calluses and removing dry, dead skin.

   ¼ cup cornmeal
   2 tablespoons liquid castile soap

Mix the cornmeal and soap in a small glass bowl until you have a paste. Massage into feet, concentrating on particularly rough spots such as the heels. Rinse with warm water and dry well.

Enzyme Ecstasy   YIELD: 1 application
Fruit acids gently exfoliate while cinnamon and mint perk up tired tootsies.

   2 drops cinnamon extract
   ¼ cup fresh pineapple, cubed
   ¼ cup fresh papaya, cubed
   5 drops peppermint essential oil

Combine the ingredients in a blender and puree until smooth. Apply the mixture to the tops and soles of the feet, and then cover with large plastic bags. Secure the bags loosely with rubber bands and put your feet up for 10 minutes. Rinse feet clean with tepid water.

Green Goddess Foot Mask   YIELD: 1 application

When avocados are in season, pamper feet with this simple moisturizing treatment.

    1 very ripe avocado, peeled and pitted

Mash the avocado to a smooth paste. Apply to the tops and soles of the feet. Cover with plastic bags, followed by white cotton socks, and leave on overnight. Rinse feet clean with tepid water.

Heavy-Duty Herbal Foot Moisturizer   YIELD: 8 ounces

Slather on this rich cream every day to keep feet soft and silky.

    ¼ cup lavender flowers
    1 tablespoon slippery elm
    ½ cup hot, not boiling, distilled water
    2 tablespoons beeswax, grated
    1 tablespoon aloe vera gel
    ½ cup almond oil
    1 teaspoon liquid vitamin E

Place the lavender and slippery elm in a glass bowl, crushing the herbs gently with the back of a wooden spoon. Cover with the water and allow to steep overnight. Strain the liquid into a glass container and set aside. Discard the plant material. In a small double boiler over medium heat, combine the beeswax, aloe, and almond oil, stirring constantly until the beeswax has melted. Add the reserved liquid and stir to mix. Remove from heat and cool slightly. Mix in the vitamin E and stir gently until well blended. Cool completely and pour into a sterilized glass jar with a tight-fitting lid. Massage into feet, concentrating on particularly rough spots.

Spicy Warming Foot Oil   YIELD: 8 ounces

Frigid feet can be miserable. Warm them quickly with this spice-scented oil.

    1 cup almond oil
    10 drops clove essential oil
    5 drops cinnamon extract

Place the ingredients in a glass jar with a tight-fitting lid. Shake well to blend. To use, massage vigorously into feet.

Summer Foot Saver   YIELD: 1 application

After being trapped in tennis shoes on a hot summer day, your feet deserve a quick cooldown. Relieve hot, itchy feet with this cooling gel.

> 5 tablespoons aloe vera gel
> 5 drops peppermint essential oil
> 5 drops eucalyptus essential oil

Combine the ingredients in a small glass bowl, whisking to blend well. Massage into feet until absorbed, concentrating on especially painful spots.

Invigorating Foot Bath   YIELD: 1 application

A day spent walking or standing can be a killer. Rest and rejuvenate sore feet with this hot herbal soak.

> ½ cup fresh peppermint, crushed
> ¼ cup fresh thyme, crushed
> ¼ cup fresh marjoram, crushed
> 2 quarts boiling distilled water

Combine the peppermint, thyme, and marjoram in a large square of cheesecloth and secure with a rubber band. Place in the bottom of a large tub and cover with the boiling water. Allow to steep until the water is comfortably warm. Remove the herbal packet and discard. Soak feet in the herbal solution for 20 minutes. Gently pat feet dry and follow with a natural moisturizer.

Oatmeal Foot Bath   YIELD: 1 application

Natural moisturizers combine with relaxing aromatherapy to soothe and smooth overworked feet.

> ½ cup oatmeal
> 2 quarts boiling distilled water
> ½ cup aloe vera gel
> 5 drops lavender essential oil

Place the oatmeal in a large square of cheesecloth and secure with a rubber band. Place in the bottom of a large tub and cover with the boiling water. Add the aloe vera gel and the lavender essential oil and stir to dissolve. Allow to steep until the water is comfortably warm. Soak feet 20 minutes, occasionally rubbing them across the oatmeal packet. Gently pat feet dry and follow with a natural moisturizer.

Sweet Feet Powder
YIELD: 12 ounces

Banish foot odor with this talc-free powder. An extra bonus: the horsetail helps stem excess perspiration.

1 cup baking soda
⅛ cup dried horsetail, finely ground
¼ cup dried chamomile, finely ground
⅛ cup dried sage, finely ground
10 drops lavender essential oil

Combine the ingredients in a small glass bowl. Stir well to evenly distribute the essential oil. Pour into a decorative glass bottle with a shaker top. To use, sprinkle liberally on feet after bathing. For greater protection, shake a bit inside shoes.

Athlete's Foot Fix
YIELD: 2 ounces

Tea tree oil and garlic are both potent antifungals in the war against athlete's foot. Like most other fungal infections, athlete's foot thrives in dark, damp environments. To keep the fungus from spreading, keep feet clean and dry, especially between the toes.

1 teaspoon tea tree oil
½ teaspoon garlic oil
¼ cup pau d'arco tea

Combine the ingredients in a small glass bottle with a tight-fitting lid. Shake well to mix. Apply to infected areas with a cotton swab several times a day.

❧ Smart Shopping ☙

Think that going natural means you must forgo indulging in pampering pedicures and manicures? Think again! Whether you treat yourself to a day at the spa or prefer to do your own hands and feet, these products can smooth, soothe, and add a dash of color.

Hand and Foot Creams

Manufacturer	Product
Aubrey Organics	Blue Green Algae Hand and Body Lotion
	Evening Primrose Lotion

	Rosa Mosqueta Lotion
	Sea Buckthorn Hand and Body Lotion
Beeswork	Nature's Lotion Hand and Body Lotion
Burt's Bees	Farmer's Friend Hand Salve
Dr. Hauschka	Hand Cream
	Rosemary Foot Balm
EO	Lemon Verbena Hand Cream
	Peppermint and Lavender Foot Balm
Jakaré	Invigorating Foot Treatment
	Softening Hand Treatment
Kettle Care	Peppermint Foot Creme
NaturElle	Bio-Active Foot Balm
Neways	Barrier Cream
Real Purity	Extra Rich Hand and Body Lotion
	Velvet Glove Hand Treatment Creme

Foot Baths

Manufacturer	*Product*
EO	Foot Salts
Mountain Rose	Feet Treat

Exfoliators

Manufacturer	*Product*
EO	Lavender and Tea Tree Foot Scrub

Foot Sprays

Manufacturer	*Product*
NaturElle	Lavender and Tea Tree Foot Spray

Foot Powders

Manufacturer	*Product*
EO	Lavender and Tea Tree Foot Powder

Cuticle Creams and Conditioners

Manufacturer	Product
Burt's Bees	Farmer's Market Lemon Butter Cuticle Creme

Nail Oils

Manufacturer	Product
Dr. Hauschka	Neem Nail Oil
Jakaré	Restoring Nail Treatment
Neways	Nail Enhancer

Nail Polish

Note: Although these nontoxic nail polishes contain no formaldehyde or toluene, some may contain chemicals that can irritate sensitive individuals.

Manufacturer	Product
Color 'N Peel	Non-Toxic Nail Polish
Earthly Delights	Earth-Friendly Nail Polish
	Liquid Bliss Nail Enamel
Nalz	Water-Based Nail Polish
Natural Beauty	Water-Based Nail Polish

Nail Polish Remover

Note: While these nontoxic nail polish removers are primarily plant based, they may not be chemical-free.

Manufacturer	Product
Earthly Delights	Naked Nails Polish Remover
No-Miss Nail Care	Almost Natural Polish Remover
Safe & Easy	Polish Remover

Nail Fungal Treatments

Manufacturer	Product
Jason	Nail Saver
ProSeed	Nail Rescue

Manicure and Pedicure Tools

Manufacturer	Product
Moom	Natural Pumice Stone
Simmons Natural	Nail Brush
Bodycare	Pedicure File
	Pumice Stone

Sing the Body Electric: Body Care

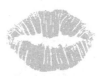

"No one can make you feel inferior without your consent."
—Eleanor Roosevelt

Nothing strikes terror in the hearts of women quite like the words *swimsuit season*. Suddenly, we focus on the condition our own bodies are in, and the thoughts are rarely flattering. Flaws, no matter how minor, jump out at us—a little pooch here, a spider vein there, the visible signs of childbirth, age spots, and, of course, the effects of gravity.

Yet, our bodies are truly miraculous and, yes, beautiful. And they are designed to last a lifetime. In order to keep our bodies at their best, we need to remember that skin care doesn't stop at the neckline. No matter what your age, shape, or size, your body needs just as much tender loving care as your face to function properly.

Dominating the world of body care is a bevy of bath and body products aimed at cleaning, smoothing, and deodorizing. Despite this abundance, the cosmetics industry has stopped short of creating cosmetics that actually protect the health of your skin. Instead, manufacturers have focused on pampering a woman's ego and soothing her senses. Products that promise to turn your bathroom into a haven from everyday stress and anxiety have become especially popular. So popular, in fact, that bath and body care products account for more than one-third of all cosmetics sales.[1]

While these products may be a delight to use, they are rarely good for your skin. Most of the products touted as spa formulas or aromatherapy treatments are overly scented with synthetic perfumes that can irritate sensitive skin. And, surprisingly, many of the high-priced bath and body treatments sold in specialty and department stores contain the same inexpensive petrochemicals and alcohols found in the cheaper drugstore brands. A good rule of thumb is to check the list of ingredients—if you wouldn't use it on your face, don't use it on your body.

Bathing Beauties

Throughout history, the bath has been used to heal, beautify, and even seduce. The ancient Egyptians bathed in expensive herbs and oils, and it's rumored that Queen Poppaea, the wife of Emperor Nero, traveled with a herd of asses to provide fresh milk for her baths.

The Romans turned bathing into an art, making it a social, spiritual, and therapeutic experience. Gathering at the public baths, noblemen and commoners alike would relax, refresh, and mingle with friends. It became such a popular indulgence that the practice soon spread throughout the world. By the dawn of the Middle Ages, however, communal bathing had become the scene of feasting, drinking, and erotic pleasures, resulting in more than a few inappropriate seductions. This outrageous behavior sparked a religious backlash that condemned all bathing as a godless pagan ritual. The church even spread rumors that exposing the body to too much water would throw it out of balance, inviting disease. Not to be dissuaded, the savvy ladies of the day simply substituted wine for the cursed bathwater.

Common folk weren't so inventive and avoided bathing like the plague, with less than healthy results. It wasn't until 1870, when Louis Pasteur made the connection between health and hygiene, that bathing regained its respectability. We've come a long way since those bath-free days. We know that cleanliness is essential to good health, and the daily bath or shower has become the norm. But in the process of getting clean, you may also be getting a tubful of toxins. Today's mainstream bath and shower products bear little resemblance to the wholesome soaps and cleansers our ancestors used.

Toxins on Tap

Whether you prefer a tubful of bubbles, bath salts, or oils, nothing can rival a hot bath after a long day for its power to relax and rejuvenate. The Greek physician Hippocrates was the first to tout the therapeutic benefits of the bath—hydrotherapy soothed sore muscles, increased circulation, and reduced swelling. Taking the bath a step further, the Japanese believed that bathing could also balance the spirit.

A good long soak is still popular today, with more than half of all women using the bath to boost their health and well-being. Unfortunately, modern bath potions could be undermining their good intentions.

Fragrant, sumptuous bath oils are a favorite addition to many baths. According to the cosmetics industry, using a bath oil will pamper your skin with richly scented oils designed to soften and moisturize. But the truth isn't quite so sensuous. Conventional nonfoaming bath oils are usually based on an inexpensive mineral or vegetable oil combined with a surfactant, which helps the oil spread out on the surface of the water, essentially turning your tub into a miniature oil slick. You feel softer after your bath because the oil simply coats the skin as you leave the tub. Foaming varieties also include oil but with the addition of foaming agents. A common combo is tri-ethanolamine (TEA) and sodium lauryl sulfate (SLS), which can form carcinogenic nitrosamines.

Most conventional bath oils contain high amounts of synthetic fragrance as well, along with FD&C colors, alcohol, and lanolin, which can all result in allergic reactions. Another common ingredient of bath oils, isopropyl myristate, can cause blackheads. Of greater concern are bath oils that combine isopropyl myristate with TEA. Research has shown that when the common cosmetics contaminant of TEA, n-nitrosodiethanolamine (NDELA), is added to isopropyl myristate, isopropyl myristate's absorption increases by a factor of 230.[2] Since bath oils remain on the skin for long periods, significant absorption of this potent carcinogen may occur.

Mineral-based bath salts, another popular tub addition, have been used for generations to heal a variety of ailments. But, again, there is nothing medicinal about today's mainstream bath salts. Used to scent, color, and soften bathwater, the bath salts purveyed by drug and department stores are based on sodium chloride, better known as common table salt. Although not toxic, sodium chloride can draw water from the skin, causing dryness. More to the point, what manufacturers do with this nontoxic ingredient may not be so benign. Synthetic dyes, perfumes, and alcohol are sprayed on the salt to create those beautiful jars of scented bath salts. Another ingredient in some bath salts is sodium sesquicarbonate, a highly alkaline chemical that can irritate the skin and mucous membranes. Borax and boric acid, both derivatives of boron, are other ingredients commonly added to bath salts to enhance the water-softening properties of the product. While both of these are toxic, a study by the University of California, San Francisco, determined that the amount of borax and boric acid absorbed by uninjured skin is very low. However, the study's researchers noted that this finding does not apply to damaged skin.[3] In 1992, the Food and Drug Administration (FDA) issued a notice stating that boric acid has not been shown safe and effective in over-the-counter products.[4]

And then there are bubbles. Nothing evokes luxury like sinking into a fragrant cloud of white foam. Then again, bubble baths, which can be purchased as either a powder or a liquid, can dry skin. Full of harsh detergents such as alkyl benzene sulfonate and irritants such as sodium tripolyphosphate, bubble baths can also cause inflammation. SLS is a common ingredient in powdered bubble baths, used as a detergent and wetting agent. Liquid bubble bath usually contains TEA-dodecylbenzene sulfonate and parabens. In addition, both types are packed with synthetic colors and fragrances, which can irritate the vaginal area. The FDA has received consumer complaints associated with bubble bath use ranging from skin irritation to urinary and bladder infections to toxic encephalopathy with brain damage.[5]

Synthetic Showers

While taking a long, luxurious bath can be a real treat, most women rely on a daily shower to keep clean. Here we enter the world of scented body washes and foaming shower gels. Although these products effectively wash away dirt and impurities, they too rely on detergents such as SLS to get the job done. An irritant that can result in dryness, roughness, and a reduction in the skin's normal barrier function, SLS is the most common ingredient in liquid soaps.

Formulated much like shampoo, body washes and shower gels also contain diethanolamine (DEA) as well as TEA. The National Toxicology Program has found that DEA, by itself, is a potent carcinogen; when these surfactants are combined with SLS, cancer-causing nitrosamines can be formed.

Virtually all mainstream cleansers also contain synthetic colors, fragrances, and preservatives to make them more attractive to consumers. Synthetic FD&C and D&C colors have been shown to cause cancer in animals. And, as you will see in the next chapter, synthetic fragrances are one of the leading causes of allergy, sensitization, and irritation. To keep the cleanser fresh for months on end, the popular parabens are added, as are other preservatives such as BHT, which can cause contact dermatitis, and tetrasodium EDTA, another ingredient that may contribute to nitrosamine formation.

Although an expanding group of bath and shower products market themselves as "spa-inspired therapy" and flaunt an assortment of botanicals, the truth is that there's nothing therapeutic about these conventional products. Since they are short on healing herbs and natural moisturizers and long on synthetic chemicals, adding these tempting tub accessories to your bath or shower routine is no better than using a bit of vegetable oil or a capful of dishwashing liquid! There is a better way.

Bath Basics

Hippocrates believed "The way to health is to have an aromatic bath every day." A hot bath can pamper your skin, whisk away stress, and even heal. Water temperature is critical. Comfortably warm water, no hotter than 108°F, softens the collagen in your joints, muscles, and membranes, and allows the healing properties of any herbs, oils, or minerals you've added to be absorbed by your skin. Anything above this temperature can increase your heart rate and the risk of scalding sensitive skin.

The beneficial properties of mineral salts come alive in a warm bath. Often used to treat swelling and inflammation, bathing in mineral salts helps detoxify your body by drawing impurities out of your skin. Mineral salts are also rich in skin-friendly trace elements. One of the most popular natural mineral salts on the market is Dead Sea salts. Containing the highest concentration of minerals on Earth, Dead Sea salts provide significant amounts of magnesium, potassium, calcium, and iodine to soothe sore muscles. A far less expensive option is Epsom salts. Made of magnesium sulfate, Epsom salts induce detoxification by promoting heavy perspiration. Epsom salts can also soothe sore muscles and soften the skin and are fragrance-free, making them particularly good for sensitive bathers. To put this cure to work for you, add two cups of mineral salts after you have filled the tub, and allow a few minutes for them to dissolve before slipping into the water.

Some women love the feel of their skin after soaking in a tub with bath oil. As you step out of the bathwater, your entire body is lightly coated with the softening oil. If the experience appeals to you, instead of floating petroleum-based oils in your bath, opt for pure plant oils such as almond, avocado, or sesame oil, which actually benefit the skin. Look for a preservative-free cold-pressed oil, and store it in your refrigerator to prevent the oil from becoming rancid. Whichever type of oil you choose, fill the tub before adding. Swirl about ¼ cup of the oil into the water to disperse it evenly over the surface.

The healing essences of herbs and essential oils can turn your bath into a healing experience. Working their magic as they enter your body through your pores and sense of smell, different herbs and essential oils can have specific effects on your body and your mind. Lavender can calm frazzled emotions and heal damaged skin, peppermint and lemongrass can revive both body and spirit after a grueling day, and chamomile can chase away insomnia. Herbs, either dried or fresh, can be added to your bath as you fill the tub. Wrap them in a square of cheesecloth tied with ribbon or string, to prevent the plant material from clogging the drain. Using essential oils instead of their herbal counterparts will give you both the herbs' healing properties and the benefit of a bath oil. Dilute essential oils in a carrier oil such as grape seed or almond oil before adding to the bath, and swirl the oils into the water to disperse them evenly. A word of warning: If you are pregnant, avoid using products that contain angelica, comfrey, feverfew, pennyroyal, sage, or yarrow.

For super skin softening, add a handful of oatmeal, barley, or bran that has been wrapped in cheesecloth to the bathwater. Along with soothing dry, chapped skin, you can use the cheesecloth bundle instead of a washcloth to gently exfoliate rough spots.

Although bubble baths can't provide tub-time therapy any more than scrubbing bubbles can clean your bathroom, if you must indulge in a cloud of bubbles, forget the irritating brands offered by cosmetics companies. Instead, pour a capful of an all-natural baby shampoo under the running water. For fragrant bubbles, add a few drops of your favorite essential oil to the shampoo.

Once your bathwater has been prepared, set aside at least twenty minutes for your soak—it takes that long for the healing properties of mineral salts or essential oils to work. But, be aware that after a half hour, the water can actually suck the moisture out of your skin.

When your time is up, exit the bath slowly, and dry off by gently pressing a soft towel over your skin. Apply a good moisturizer or body lotion while your skin is still damp to boost its effectiveness.

The Sensuous Soak

Turkish women of old knew how to turn an ordinary bath into a pampering ritual. Visiting the famed Turkish baths, or *hamam*, a woman would take up to twenty bath accessories with her. Along with the traditional soap and towel, or *pestemal*, a *hamam* bundle might include a silver bowl for pouring water over the body, a smaller bowl for henna, a *kese* mitt to massage and exfoliate, and a vial of attar of rose, the only fragrance considered proper for a newly washed body.[6]

Indulge yourself with your own *hamam* kit and include a long-handle bath brush, a comfy bath pillow, a loofah or exfoliating bath mitt, and your favorite essential oils. Place them in a pretty basket next to the tub, or set them out on a bath tray.

For the maximum therapeutic experience, light a candle or two and put on some soft, soothing music before you slide into the tub. Support your head with a bath pillow, stretch out, and take deep, slow breaths to fully absorb the steamy scents. To totally unwind, tighten each muscle group, beginning with the toes and progressing slowly to your head, relaxing each in turn.

Shower Power

While we all love the indulgence of a pampering bath, there are times when a five-minute shower is all you can carve out of your busy schedule. Fortunately, you can turn your shower into a naturally pleasant experience without relying on potentially dangerous cleansers.

Despite all the new shower products cluttering store shelves, soap seems to be a staple among the shower brigade. However, traditional soaps can be drying, and the new breed of moisturizing and deodorizing "soaps" can turn your shower into a chemical stew. Glycerin and olive oil–based castile soaps, available in either bar or liquid form, are mild alternatives to harsh, potentially harmful soaps. For silky smooth skin, look for products containing emollient-rich avocado, almond, or jojoba oil. Honey is another ingredient with excellent moisturizing properties. For a nourishing treat, choose a soap with hemp seed oil. Highly moisturizing and mildly antiseptic, hemp is rich in essential fatty acids, as well as vitamins A, C, D, and E and the B vitamins.

Natural body washes and shower gels containing herbal essential oils can also pamper the skin. Aloe vera, rose, or chamomile will soothe delicate dry skin. Oily skin may benefit from frankincense or lemon essential oil. The addition of herbal essential oils can also turn your shower into an aromatherapeutic spa. To rejuvenate and energize, try a castile-based soap with citrus, geranium, or mint. Stressed out? Choose a product with lavender or cedar essential oil to wash away frazzled nerves. And ylang-ylang or patchouli will leave you feeling sensuous and beautiful.

Tub Tools

Most of us grew up bathing or showering armed with only a bar of soap and a washcloth. While these tools can effectively keep you clean, today's natural-bath market offers so much more! Boost your bathing experience with one or more of the following bath accessories:

Loofahs
Soft and pliable when wet, these natural vegetable sponges exfoliate the skin and stimulate circulation. Gently scrubbing your skin with a loofah in the shower or bath will remove dead skin cells and impurities.

Sisal Cloths
Taking a twist on the traditional washcloth, sisal cloths are also derived from vegetable fibers. Available formats include washcloths, body gloves, and back straps. Washing with sisal boosts the body's natural detoxification process by stimulating the lymphatic and circulatory systems.

Sea Sponges
More durable and absorbent than synthetic bath sponges, sea sponges resist stains and odors, due to an intricate system of canals. Less abrasive than loofahs or sisal cloths, sea sponges are ideal for damaged or sensitive skin. They come in a variety of sizes, shapes, and textures.

Natural-Bristle Bath Brushes
There's one available for just about every part of your body. Long-handle models can scrub your back, while short-handle or handheld varieties are great for cleaning your arms, legs, and torso.

Whichever tools you use, clean them in hot, soapy water often to prevent mold, mildew, and bacteria from forming.

Stimulating Strokes

Women with naturally glowing skin share a secret known simply as skin brushing. Ridiculously inexpensive, it's one beauty treatment that isn't advertised in magazines or promoted in most beauty books. But it's essential for creating beautifully healthy skin.

Skin brushing is a simple way to stimulate circulation of the small capillaries just below the surface of the skin. A daily brushing also helps eliminate wastes and keeps skin smooth by removing dead skin cells. Skin brushing is best done right before showering so that you can wash away all of the exfoliated skin and waste products.

Using a dry, natural-bristle brush, begin by brushing your feet, and work your way up over your legs, torso, and arms, using smooth, upward strokes. Do not brush your face, your breasts, or any area that is tender or inflamed since the bristles can irritate delicate skin. Once you get the hang of skin brushing, the whole treatment shouldn't take more than five minutes. After a few months of brushing your skin every day, you'll notice a definite difference in its appearance and texture.

Body Smoothers

If you check the labels on most body lotions, you'll find they contain many of the same ingredients as mainstream hand lotions and moisturizers. Not surprisingly, conventional products are filled with petrochemicals such as petrolatum or mineral oil, which can clog pores and lead to blemishes. Surfactants, such as TEA, are included as wetting agents to allow the product to penetrate the skin more easily. Preservative-heavy, these body lotions also contain formaldehyde releasers such as DMDM hydantoin and quaternium-15 or any of the potentially hormone-disrupting parabens.

Although these products are promoted as overall moisturizers, occasionally a company will come out with a cream supposedly designed to address a specific problem. Among the most popular are cellulite creams. Cellulite is a result of unevenly distributed fatty tissue that usually targets the thighs, hips, and buttocks. Widely regarded as genetic, cellulite often appears after a woman's thirtieth birthday, particularly if the woman is overweight.

Some health professionals don't buy the argument that you inherit the propensity of developing cellulite, often labeled "orange-peel skin" or "cottage-cheese thighs." Instead, they believe cellulite is a result of a poor diet, a sedentary lifestyle, and poor elimination and circulation. According to their theory, when circulation and elimination are sluggish, toxins in the bloodstream become trapped in the fat cells, creating that puckered look.

Unfortunately, there is no cure for cellulite. Mainstream cellulite creams are usually nothing more than traditional moisturizers with the addition of "cellulite-fighting compounds," such as alpha hydroxy acids or caffeine. Despite their claims, these products are simply another example of hope in a bottle. What's more, a study by the Finnish Institute of Occupational Health found that cellulite creams contain a large number of ingredients, 25 percent of which have been shown to cause allergic reactions.[7]

Even though these miracle creams do nothing to eradicate the problem, you don't have to take cellulite lying down. Since extra pounds and poor muscle tone can make the problem worse, adopting a healthy diet and exercise routine can lessen the appearance of cellulite. And skin brushing can help reduce the cottage-cheese effect temporarily by boosting circulation. Massaging trouble spots can also stimulate both the circulatory and the lymphatic systems, which is reported to help break down fat and eliminate wastes and toxins.

A Close Shave

Your body can be trim, your skin glowing—but the picture isn't complete if your legs and underarms sport stubble. For the vast majority of women—about 90 percent—that means wielding a razor an average of three times a week.

Women have been shaving away unwanted hair for centuries—ever since 400 B.C. But shaving didn't become a widely practiced ritual until an advertising campaign in 1915 convinced American women that excess hair was unhygienic and unfeminine. Shaving has become so much a part of our beauty routine that we wouldn't dream of letting our leg and underarm hair grow au naturel.

While shaving can leave your legs, underarms, and bikini line smooth and hair-free, it's a practice with its fair share of pitfalls. Nicks, razor burns, and unsightly red bumps are common. Shaving with an electric razor can leave you with dry, flaky skin, as can lathering up with soap and water. What's a girl to do? According to manufacturers of personal care products, a shaving cream or gel can save you from the irritating consequences of shaving. Full of rich, creamy lather and good-for-you ingredients such as aloe vera and vitamin E, these products promise a smooth shave that will leave you with silky soft skin. One product even contains "microbeads" to exfoliate skin as you shave. But before you reach for your razor, let's look at what's really in your shaving cream.

Drugstore shaving creams and gels may produce mountains of luscious lather, but that lather comes with a price. Home to an amazing number of ingredients, today's shaving preparations are based largely on synthetic chemicals, with a smattering of botanicals to enhance marketability. The rich foaming qualities that are the hallmark of these products usually come from some combination of TEA, lauramide DEA, and sarcosines, a foaming agent found in starfish and sea urchins.[8] Solvents are also included to aid in the product's function. One solvent widely used in shaving gels is isopentane, a flammable hydrocarbon derived from petroleum, which can irritate the skin. To soften skin, emollients such as mineral oil, propylene glycol, and lanolin are also included. Polyvinylpyrrolidone (PVP), a contact allergen, gives the cream or gel body.

Lest you confuse these new feminine products with your husband's shaving cream, FD&C colors are added to lend a delicate pink, blue, or lavender hue to the product. To make the experience truly pampering, manufacturers also include synthetic fragrance. In fact, one well-known brand of shaving gel lists fragrance eleventh out of the thirty ingredients in the product. (Remember, ingredients are listed in descending order of prevalence.)

Preservatives are also customary additions to shaving formulas and can include any or all of the following: DMDM hydantoin; polyquaternium-10, a water-soluble antimicrobial that may be a formaldehyde releaser and sensitizer; methylchloroisothiazolinone/methylisothiazolinone, a skin-sensitizing, moderately toxic broad-spectrum preservative; and iodopropynl butylcarbamate (IPBC). Researchers at the University of Copenhagen in Denmark have identified IPBC as a contact allergen.[9] Although the Cosmetic Ingredient Review Panel considers IPBC safe in concentrations up to 0.1 percent, the panel advises that this preservative should not be used in aerosol products.[10]

Taking the lead from men's shaving creams, these products are pressurized and rely on petroleum-derived butane or propane as propellants. Even shaving gels, which would be just as effective if packaged in a pump or tube, contain these propellants. Although safe if used by consumers as directed, both ingredients are highly flammable and may cause an explosion and fire when stored improperly.

If you aren't ready to give up your razor but don't want to expose yourself to harmful shaving creams and gels, here are some steps you can take to ensure a smooth shave without resorting to chemical creams and gels:

1. Don't shave first thing in the morning since body fluids retained during the night tend to make the skin puffy. Wait at least a half hour, to allow your skin to normalize.
2. Use a clean, sharp blade. Dull blades require more force to cut hair and can increase the chance of nicks and cuts.
3. For best results, soak the skin to be shaved in warm water for at least five minutes.
4. Aloe vera gel is an effective skin-softening alternative to mainstream shaving gels. Simply smooth a thick coating of gel on your legs, and shave as usual. An added benefit: aloe vera also possesses anti-inflammatory properties.
5. Use long, smooth strokes when shaving your legs, and shave in the opposite direction from which the hair grows. Rinse the razor after each stroke to remove hair and dead skin cells.
6. To avoid irritation, don't revisit an area that's already been shaved.
7. Wait several hours or overnight to apply a deodorant or antiperspirant (even a natural one) to underarms. Using astringents and antiseptic ingredients on freshly shaved underarms can sting and cause irritation.
8. After shaving, dry off by gently patting the area with a soft, absorbent towel. Smooth legs and/or bikini area with another dose of aloe vera gel or a natural moisturizer to soothe any irritation and prevent dryness.

Deadly Depilatories

Long before the advent of safety razors, women whisked away unwanted hair with homemade depilatory creams. Concocted by mixing arsenic, quicklime, and starch, these depilatories could easily have given new meaning to the term *killer legs*.

By A.D. 54, using depilatories had become a trend among well-to-do women, who relied on the latest technology to stay fuzz-free—a mixture of resin, pitch, ivy gum, asses fat, she-goat gall, bat's blood, and powdered viper. While these ingredients may sound bizarre and potentially lethal, modern depilatories may not be much safer.

Today's depilatories remove hair below the surface of the skin by dissolving it with a high-pH chemical. Originally, hydrogen sulfide was the chemical of choice. Although highly effective, sulfides have a strong, unpleasant odor that made consumers curl up their noses. So, manufacturers switched to thioglycolic acid, which smells slightly less offensive but still dissolves hair. But thioglycolates, too, have their drawbacks, including skin irritation, severe allergic reactions, and pustular outbreaks. Since thioglycolates don't remove hair as well as sulfides, calcium hydroxide (lye) is often added to modern depilatories to boost the products' effectiveness—an addition that can burn the skin and eyes. Strong perfumes are also added to mask thioglycolates' unpleasant odor.

Depilatories are available in creams, lotions, mousses, gels, and even roll-ons. Regardless of the form, to work effectively, depilatories must remain on the skin for as long as fifteen minutes, during which time they burrow into the pores with chemicals that not only destroy hair but can damage skin as well.

Waxing Poetic

Waxing is second only to shaving as the popular choice for removing unwanted hair. Waxing first gained attention when salons across America began offering this service as a way to banish hair from the face and legs. How does waxing work? The hot wax, usually made from rosin, beeswax, or paraffin, is spread over the area where hair is to be removed and covered with a strip of muslin. As the wax cools, it hardens around each hair. The strip is then ripped off, taking the hair with it. While not particularly toxic, the process can be painful.

Why do women wax? Despite the pain, waxing produces smoother results that last for four to six weeks, instead of the typical two to three days experienced with shaving. But waxing can cause damage, producing tissue trauma and leaving you with highly tender, bright red skin, a condition that can persist for hours. Scabbing and welts are also common side effects of this uncomfortable process.

If you must wax, avoid doing so during the three days prior to the onset of your menstrual cycle and also the following three days since your skin is more sensitive during that time of the month. Also—and this should go without saying—never wax sunburned skin. To reduce the amount of redness, use a lavender- or calendula-based moisturizer or an aloe vera gel immediately after waxing.

A less painful way to remove hair is with the ancient art of sugaring. The process, which originated in Egypt thousands of years ago, uses a thick sugar- and water-based gel to remove hair. Unlike hot wax, the sugar is gently warmed, reducing the chance of burns. Better yet, the sugaring gel adheres only to the hair and not the skin, so the "ouch" factor is less of an issue. And since you are using a gel instead of a wax, residue can be gently wiped away with a soft washcloth dampened in warm water.

Though sugaring was once offered only in salons, sugaring kits are now available for home use. But before you buy, check the label. Unlike natural sugaring kits, which contain only sugar, water, and herbs, some drugstore varieties add parabens, imidazolidinyl urea, and FD&C colors, which may promote contact dermatitis.

Lose It with Lasers

The newest tool in the hair-removal game is a technique that uses lasers to zap unwanted hair. The technique works by passing light through the skin, where it is absorbed by the melanin in the hair follicles. Over the next two months, the hair gradually falls out. Although no one knows exactly why lasers have this effect on the hair, a popular theory is that the intense heat generated by the laser destroys the hair follicle.

Before you rush out to your nearest laser clinic, be aware that the FDA does not allow manufacturers to claim that their lasers offer permanent results.[11] Although the process can reduce the amount of hair you have and decrease its thickness, it's not a permanent solution. It's also expensive and time-consuming. Removing the hair on just one leg can cost between $500 and $1,000.[12] Three to four treatments, six to eight weeks apart, may be needed before you see a meaningful reduction in the amount of hair you have. What's more, it's not terribly effective on people with light-color hair or on those with dark complexions. Also, no matter how high-tech the treatment seems, it's not without side effects. The area treated will be sensitive and may be swollen and red. More-serious skin reactions can include peeling, blistering, and burning as well as dark patches or a loss of pigment.

Electric Shock

Electrolysis is the only permanent method of hair removal approved by the FDA. Unlike laser treatments, which target large areas at once, electrolysis treats each hair individually. A needle epilator injects a fine wire probe into the hair follicle. An electric current travels down the wire and destroys the papilla (the area at the base of the follicle that produces hair). The loosened hair is then removed with the aid of tweezers specifically designed for electrolysis. Although electrolysis is permanent, it isn't an overnight cure for unwanted hair. To get satisfactory results, you may be required to commit to frequent treatments over the course of a few months to perhaps a year or more.

Although most dermatologists use well-maintained equipment and disposable needles, salon-based electrologists may not. Risks include electric shock from poorly insulated equipment, infection from unsterilized needles, and scarring from use of improper technique. Finding a qualified practitioner may also be a problem since there are no uniform standards for licensing.

If you don't want to invest the time and money in professional electrolysis, you may be tempted by one of the home electrolysis kits advertised on late-night infomercials. While these devices may work in theory, they require a high level of skill to properly exterminate unwanted hair. If the angle and depth are not completely accurate when the probe is inserted, you may damage your skin. Burns, pitting, and scarring are common complaints from home users. Moreover, a shallow insertion can cauterize the upper follicle and seal the hair under the skin's surface, a condition that can lead to infection. For do-it-yourself types, it's much safer to stick with the less damaging methods of hair removal.

Sweating the Small Stuff

At the first inkling of wetness, we panic. Whether it's from the heat or just a bad case of nerves, perspiration can often lead to body odor. To guard against becoming odorous social outcasts, we spray, powder, and perfume ourselves with all sorts of chemical deodorants and antiperspirants.

Staying fresh and odor-free has become an American obsession—one that manufacturers have parlayed into a $1.4 billion market.[13] It hasn't always been so. The first commercial deodorant was developed in 1888, but it wasn't until after World War II that the idea of preventing body odor captured America's attention. Our postwar love affair with modern science, coupled with slick advertising, made deodorants and antiperspirants a staple in medicine cabinets across the country.

Even though we may think of perspiration as an embarrassing nuisance, our bodies couldn't survive without it. It's one of the methods the body uses to eliminate toxins from the system. And when we are overheated, perspiration regulates our body temperature, cooling us as the moisture evaporates.

In fact, body odor, too, may serve a purpose. Since human body odor develops during adolescence, some researchers believe that naturally produced scents contain pheromones, chemicals that contribute to sexual attraction. According to James Duke, Ph.D., author of *The Green Pharmacy*, "Scientists have known for a long time that pheromones play a principal role in animal mating. But until fairly recently, conventional scientific wisdom held that these chemicals had no amorous effect on us humans. Now studies have demonstrated that pheromones do indeed play a subtle, but very real, role in human attraction."[14] Indeed, each of us has our own particular scent. But when our individual aroma becomes a bit more than pleasing, it's time to take action.

You don't have to be a marathon runner to have a problem with excess sweat and body odor. Sweat glands—millions of them—cover our skin, secreting up to six cups of moisture per day. Although we normally don't notice this constant process, when the weather turns hot and humid, that amount can easily increase to seventeen cups! No wonder we're left feeling like a wet dishrag.

Our bodies contain two types of sweat glands—eccrine and apocrine. The eccrine glands act as the body's thermostat, and the sweat they produce is virtually odorless. The apocrine glands, on the other hand, produce body odor and are located under the arms, around the nipples, and in the genital area. However, the sweat that apocrine glands produce, which is mainly salt water, isn't the culprit. The problem is the bacteria that lives on the surface of the skin and feeds on our perspiration. The bacteria gobbles up the moisture, decomposes it, and causes odor.

While an unusually strong odor might be a social embarrassment, some health care practitioners believe that it can also be an indication of illness.

The theory is that an unpleasant odor is a signal that something is out of balance. For example, a rancid odor could point to an imbalance in the liver and small intestine, diabetes, or a yeast infection.

"The type of foods you eat can also contribute to the way you smell," says Elson Haas, M.D., founder and director of the Preventive Medical Center of Marin in San Rafael, California, and author of *The Detox Diet* and *Staying Healthy with Nutrition*. He adds, "A meat-based diet makes a person more prone to body odor." While eating animal products may contribute to the problem, vegetarians aren't immune. Garlic, curry, and highly spiced foods contain volatile oils that, when mixed with sweat, can be potent. If you're hooked on a spicy diet, Dr. Haas suggests adding an edible deodorant, such as parsley, oregano, papaya, or cinnamon, to your cuisine.[15]

The Protection Racket

Both deodorants and antiperspirants fight odor, but they work very differently on the body. Deodorants simply inhibit the growth of bacteria that causes odor, while antiperspirants stop perspiration by blocking the pores. The dissimilarity in the two products' actions is reflected in how the FDA classifies them: deodorants are considered cosmetics because they work only on the skin's surface; antiperspirants are treated as over-the-counter drugs because they change how the body functions. Each product has its drawbacks; the synthetic chemicals found in conventional deodorants and antiperspirants may pose health threats, especially to chemically sensitive users.

Using a perfumed base, deodorants contain antiseptic and antibacterial ingredients, such as triclosan, that control bacterial decomposition and inhibit the growth of microorganisms. To have any lasting effect, this type of product must remain in the pores.

Conventional deodorants also rely on quaternary ammonium compounds to waylay odor. While highly effective, quaternary ammonium compounds may be toxic, with concentrations as low as 0.1 percent irritating to the eyes and mucous membranes.[16] In addition, all synthetic deodorants can cause enlarged sweat glands, pimples under the arms, and lung and throat irritation.

Antiperspirants, on the other hand, curb wetness by temporarily shrinking the size of the sweat glands. The most common ingredients in commercial antiperspirants include aluminum salts, urea, and propylene glycol. Of these, aluminum chlorohydrate has caused the most concern. "Aluminum is a highly toxic substance in your brain," says Theo Kruck, Ph.D., associate professor of physiology (ret.) at the University of Toronto, who has participated in several studies investigating aluminum's impact on health.[17] Although controversial, these early studies have linked aluminum to the development of Alzheimer's disease, prompting some health care practitioners to speculate about the cumulative health effects of aluminum over a lifetime of exposure. But William Pendlebury, M.D., professor of pathology at the University of Vermont at Burlington, says these fears are groundless. Although no safe level of aluminum has been established, Pendlebury says, "Most of the aluminum we ingest comes from our food and water. The amount found in antiperspirants is trivial."[18] While the jury is still out on the connection between aluminum and Alzheimer's, antiperspirants can pose other health threats.

Talc is another problematic ingredient of many antiperspirants. It is used as an agent in the manufacturing process, and prolonged inhalation can cause inflammation of the lungs, bronchial irritation, and the development of fibrous lesions. To reduce these risks, avoid aerosol antiperspirant sprays. Although these products are quick and convenient, the fine mist they produce contains not only aluminum and talc particles but also petrochemical propellants that are easily inhaled.[19]

The Air Down There

Back in 1966, a new deodorant product appeared on store shelves that claimed to be "essential to your cleanliness and your peace of mind about being a girl—an attractive, nice-to-be-with girl." The labels on these feminine deodorant sprays have changed over the past three decades to reflect our changing society, but until recently, the ingredients were essentially the same. Promising to banish odor in the genital area, these products traditionally relied on talc to keep private parts fresh and dry. Chemically similar to asbestos, talc isn't associated only with respiratory problems. The fine powder has been linked to an increase in ovarian cancer in a study by the Fred Hutchinson Cancer Research Center in Seattle. Since the chemicals found in talc-based products migrate up the vaginal canal to the reproductive tract, the study found that women who used feminine deodorant sprays had an increased ovarian cancer risk of 90 percent.[20] While the two leading manufacturers of feminine deodorant sprays have switched from talc to cornstarch in response to consumer demand, other ingredients in these products remain a cause for concern.

Most prevalent are isopropyl myristate and benzyl alcohol, which is corrosive to the skin and mucous membranes. The University of Maryland, College Park, Health Center warns that these irritants can also contribute to the development of yeast infections when sprayed on underwear and sanitary pads or, as manufacturers suggest, directly on the vaginal area.[21]

While the makers of feminine deodorant sprays have gotten the message regarding talc, manufacturers of deodorant body powders haven't. Unfortunately, neither have the thousands of women who liberally sprinkle these powders under their arms and around their genitals every day.

Get Fresh Naturally

If the thought of spraying all of these chemicals under your arms and around your genitals sends you in search of healthier alternatives, rest assured that there are nontoxic defenses you can use to fight body odor. Natural deodorants rely on antibacterial herbs, such as coriander, chamomile, and lichen, which inhibit the growth of underarm bacteria. Some natural brands also include antiseptic herbs such as lavender, sage, and tea tree oil.

While some health-conscious women prefer a simple deodorant, others still like the wetness-blocking action of an antiperspirant. Botanical astringents, such as witch hazel, tighten the skin cells, reducing the amount of moisture that escapes through the pores. A dusting of cornstarch, arrowroot, or baking soda can also keep you dry.

Another alternative to conventional antiperspirants is the deodorant stone. Made from mineral salts, the stones resemble hunks of quartz. Unlike mainstream products, which clog pores and may be absorbed into the body, the fragrance-free mineral salts work on the surface of the skin to kill existing bacteria and inhibit the growth of new microbes. One stone can last up to two years, making it an economical and environmentally friendly choice.

Your choice in clothing can also help minimize wetness. Trade in ultratight jeans and panty hose for more comfortably fitting clothes. Besides contributing to skin irritations and yeast infections, skin-hugging jeans and panty hose trap perspiration in the groin area, making the area an ideal breeding ground for bacteria. Opt for natural fabrics that breathe. Cotton, hemp, and other lightweight fabrics allow the air to circulate around the body, evaporating moisture before it becomes a problem. Finally, choose light colors since darker shades absorb the heat and show perspiration stains more readily than white or light-color fabric.

Pamper your body with healing herbs for healthy, glowing skin. Look for the botanical ingredients in Table 7.1 when shopping for body care products, or try one of the herb-rich formulas at the end of this chapter for bath and body cosmetics guaranteed to rival anything a spa has to offer.

Homemade Body Care

Custom bath and body products designed for an individual's skin type are virtually unknown in the cosmetics industry. But with a little time, knowledge, and creativity, you can create the cosmetics you need to maintain soft, healthy skin from the neck down.

Bath Additives

Slipping into a tub of warm, scented water not only boosts your spirits but also can cleanse, soften, and even heal your body. Based on medicinal herbs, aromatherapeutic essential oils, and pure plant compounds, these bath formulas are good for both body and soul.

Herbal Waters   YIELD: 12 ounces
Turn your bath into a pampering spa treatment full of moisturizing plant oils and skin-friendly herbal essential oils.

   1 cup almond oil
   ½ cup avocado oil
   10 drops lavender essential oil
   8 drops chamomile essential oil
   4 drops ylang-ylang essential oil
   2 drops rose geranium essential oil

Combine the ingredients in a 12-ounce glass bottle with a lid or stopper. Close tightly and shake well to mix the oils. Store the mixture in a cool, dark place for 24 hours to allow the oils to blend. To use, add ¼ cup to your bathwater.

Table 7.1 🍃 Herbal Remedies for a Beautiful Body

If You Have . . .	Useful Herbs	Comments and Cautions
age spots	horseradish, lemon	Horseradish may irritate sensitive skin.
blemishes	burdock, calendula, garlic, lavender, lemon, nasturtium, tea tree oil	
body odor	chamomile, coriander, sage	
cellulite	ginger, horsetail, plantain, seaweed	
dry skin	chamomile, lavender, neroli, rose, rose geranium, sandalwood	
inflammation	aloe vera, chamomile, horse chestnut, witch hazel	
irritated skin	aloe vera, calendula, chamomile, lavender	
itchy skin	aloe vera, chamomile	
oily skin	cedarwood, grapefruit seed extract, lemon, sage, yarrow	
perspiration	witch hazel	
stretch marks	aloe vera, lavender	
sun-damaged skin	aloe vera, carrot seed oil, marshmallow, pau d'arco, sesame oil	

Sinfully Sensuous Bath Oil   YIELD: 1 bath

Bathing isn't just for getting clean. It's the ultimate experience in sensuality. This is the perfect bath to prepare you for an evening of romance.

½ cup almond oil
3 drops each jasmine, sandalwood, and ylang-ylang essential oils

Combine the almond oil and the essential oils, stirring well to mix. Add to a full bath; put on some soft music, and don't forget to light some candles.

Moisturizing Milk Bath   YIELD: 1 bath

Milk is the classic bathing aid to relieve dry skin.

4 cups distilled water
2 cups instant powdered milk
½ cup oatmeal (optional)
5 drops patchouli essential oil (optional)

Mix the water and powdered milk, stirring well to dissolve. Add to a tub full of warm water.

To relieve the itchiness that often accompanies dry skin, combine the oatmeal and patchouli essential oil and wrap in a square of cheesecloth. Secure the cheesecloth tightly with a string or rubber band, and use instead of a washcloth to soften, soothe, and exfoliate.

Energy Bath   YIELD: 1 bath

Use this citrus soak to revive body and spirit after a hard day.

1 tablespoon almond oil
5 drops lavender essential oil
4 drops peppermint essential oil
3 drops each grapefruit and lemongrass essential oils

Mix the ingredients thoroughly and swirl through your bathwater just before getting into the tub.

Sweet Dreams   YIELD: 1 bath

Can't sleep? Try this soothing bath just before bedtime.

1 cup chamomile flowers
8 drops lavender essential oil

Tie the chamomile into a cheesecloth bundle and secure with a string or rubber band. As the bathtub fills, place the packet under the running water. Just before climbing into the tub, add the lavender essential oil.

Detox Bath   YIELD: 1 bath
The minerals in this bath promote sweating, helping your body rid itself of toxins and environmental pollutants. To enhance detoxifying perspiration, sip a cup of herbal tea while you soak.

> 2 cups Epsom salts
> 1 cup baking soda
> 1 cup sea salt

Add the ingredients to your bathwater as you fill the tub, swirling the water with your hand to mix and dissolve the salts. To receive the full benefit of the minerals, allow yourself at least 20 minutes to soak.

Muscle-Soothing Soak   YIELD: 1 bath
Relieve everyday aches and pains with this healing herbal bath. Note: Arnica can burn the skin and should never be used unless it is diluted in a 5:1 water solution.

> 2 cups Epsom salts
> 10 drops tea tree essential oil
> 1 teaspoon arnica

As your tub fills, dissolve the Epsom salts under the running water. Just before entering the bath, add the tea tree oil and arnica, swirling to blend with the bathwater.

Sunburn Soother   YIELD: 1 bath
Although we know that ultraviolet exposure increases the risk of developing skin cancer and speeds up aging, there may be times when you find yourself with a painful sunburn. If you've overdone your solar celebration, try this herbal soother.

> ¼ cup lavender flowers
> ¼ cup calendula flowers
> ¼ cup pau d'arco
> 1 quart boiling distilled water

½ cup oatmeal

1 cup aloe vera juice

Place the lavender, calendula, and pau d'arco in a large glass bowl, and cover with the boiling water. Allow the herbs to steep for 20 minutes. Strain the herbs and discard, reserving the liquid.

Wrap the oatmeal in a square of cheesecloth and secure tightly with a string or rubber band. Place the oatmeal packet in the bottom of your tub, and draw a cool bath, allowing the water to flow over the packet. Add the reserved herbal tea and the aloe vera juice, stirring the water to mix.

Submerge as much of your body in the water as possible. Soak for at least 10 minutes. For a particularly severe burn, follow your bath by gently smoothing aloe vera gel on burned areas.

Soothing Sun Bath Vinegar   YIELD: 1 bath

Apple cider vinegar can take the sting out of the nastiest sunburn.

3 cups apple cider vinegar

10 drops lavender essential oil

Draw a cool bath. Add the vinegar and essential oil, stirring the water to mix.

Submerge as much of your body in the water as possible. Soak for at least 10 minutes. For a particularly severe burn, follow your bath by gently smoothing aloe vera gel on burned areas.

Body Cleansers

A fragrant body wash can turn your shower into an instant aromatherapy treatment. Instead of buying high-priced chemical cleansers, indulge in one of these herbal body washes.

Wake-Up Wash   YIELD: 8 ounces

The fresh scent of citrus will energize your morning shower.

1 cup liquid castile soap

1 tablespoon avocado oil

5 drops grapefruit essential oil

3 drops lemongrass essential oil

2 drops rosemary essential oil

Combine the ingredients in a plastic bottle with a tight-fitting lid. Cap and shake well to blend.

Lavender Fields   Yield: 8 ounces

Try this relaxing, lavender-scented body cleanser to wash away stress and anxiety.

> 1 cup liquid castile soap
> 1 tablespoon almond oil
> 8 drops lavender essential oil
> 3 drops ylang-ylang essential oil
> 2 drops rose essential oil

Combine the ingredients in a plastic bottle with a tight-fitting lid. Cap and shake well to blend.

Desert Essence Moisturizing Shower Gel   Yield: 8 ounces

The arid desert is home to a surprising number of natural moisturizers.

> ½ cup liquid castile soap
> ½ cup aloe vera gel
> 1 tablespoon jojoba oil
> 6 drops chamomile essential oil
> 2 drops sandalwood essential oil

Combine the ingredients in a glass bowl and stir to blend. Pour into a plastic bottle with a tight-fitting lid.

Bacteria-Fighting Body Wash   Yield: 8 ounces

This body wash has deodorizing properties to eliminate the bacteria that cause body odor.

> 1 cup liquid castile soap
> 1 tablespoon witch hazel
> 4 drops chamomile essential oil
> 4 drops sage essential oil
> 2 drops tea tree oil
> 2 drops rose geranium essential oil

Combine the ingredients in a plastic bottle with a tight-fitting lid. Cap and shake well to blend.

Body Scrubs

When it comes to exfoliating, don't stop at your face! These body scrubs can whisk away dead skin cells and leave you with radiant skin all over.

Body Buffer   YIELD: 5 ounces
This gentle, orange-scented scrub will remove dead skin cells and impurities while you shower.

> ½ cup aloe vera gel
> 2 tablespoons cornmeal
> 2 drops neroli essential oil

Combine the aloe vera and cornmeal in a small plastic bowl, stirring well to blend. Mix in the essential oil. To use, massage the scrub all over your body, concentrating on rough spots such as heels and elbows. Rinse and pat your skin dry.

Herbal Salt Scrub   YIELD: 12 ounces
Get your body glowing with this spa-inspired herbal scrub. The plant oils soften your skin while the sea salt stimulates circulation.

> 1 cup coarse sea salt
> ¼ cup almond oil
> ¼ cup sesame oil
> 1 teaspoon liquid vitamin E
> 1 tablespoon chamomile flowers, crushed
> 1 tablespoon lavender flowers, crushed

Mix the ingredients in a glass bowl. Spoon the mixture into a clean plastic jar with a tight-fitting lid. Cap and store in a cool, dark place for 24 hours to allow the ingredients to blend. To use, massage the scrub all over your body, concentrating on rough spots such as heels and elbows. Rinse and pat your skin dry.

Body Lotions

Applying a moisturizer to your body is every bit as important as moisturizing your face. A daily dose of body lotion will help keep your skin healthy and velvety soft.

Chocolate-Mint Body Smoother   YIELD: 4 ounces

Emollient-rich cocoa butter has a delicious chocolate scent. Combined with mint, this light lotion is a treat for both the body and the senses.

2 ounces cocoa butter
¼ cup apricot kernel oil
1 teaspoon beeswax, grated
1 teaspoon liquid vitamin E
3 drops peppermint essential oil

Combine the cocoa butter, apricot oil, and beeswax in a small saucepan. Heat on low until the cocoa butter and beeswax have completely melted. Remove from heat and cool slightly. Add the vitamin E and peppermint essential oil, stirring well to blend. Pour into a clean container and allow to cool completely before capping with a tight-fitting lid.

Soothing Herbal Body Lotion   YIELD: 8 ounces

Skin-friendly herbs combine with moisturizing plant oils to soften and heal dry, neglected skin.

1 teaspoon dried lavender flowers
1 teaspoon dried calendula flowers
1 teaspoon dried chamomile flowers
½ cup boiling distilled water
1 teaspoon beeswax, grated
¼ cup avocado oil
¼ cup wheat germ oil
½ teaspoon liquid vitamin E
½ teaspoon liquid vitamin C
3 drops rose essential oil

Bundle the lavender, calendula, and chamomile in a square of cheesecloth and secure with a string or rubber band. Pour the boiling water over the packet and allow to steep for 20 minutes. Remove the packet and discard, reserving the liquid.

Melt the beeswax in the top of a double boiler. Slowly add the avocado and wheat germ oils, stirring constantly with a wooden spoon until incorporated. Remove the mixture from the heat, and slowly add the reserved herbal infusion, stirring until well blended. Cool slightly, and add the vitamins E and C and the essential oil, mixing well. Pour into a clean bottle. Cool and cap tightly.

Citrus Zinger Body Lotion

YIELD: 8 ounces

Just because you have oily skin, don't think you can forget about your body's need for moisture. This lotion provides moisture while controlling excess oil, thanks to its astringent herbs.

    1 teaspoon dried yarrow
    ½ cup boiling distilled water
    2 tablespoons witch hazel
    ¼ cup aloe vera gel
    1 teaspoon beeswax, grated
    ¼ cup jojoba oil
    ½ teaspoon liquid vitamin E
    ½ teaspoon liquid vitamin C
    ½ teaspoon grapefruit seed extract
    3 drops lemon essential oil

Wrap the yarrow in a square of cheesecloth and secure with a string or rubber band. Place the packet in a small bowl, pour the boiling water over it, and allow to steep for 20 minutes. Remove the packet and discard. Add the witch hazel and aloe to the warm infusion, and stir to mix.

Melt the beeswax in the top of a double boiler. Slowly add the jojoba oil, stirring constantly with a wooden spoon until incorporated. Remove the mixture from the heat and slowly add the reserved herbal infusion, stirring until well blended. Cool slightly and add the vitamins E and C, the grapefruit seed extract, and the essential oil, mixing well. Pour into a clean bottle. Cool and cap tightly.

Sun Repair in a Bottle

YIELD: 8 ounces

Studies show that aloe vera and vitamin E actually help repair sun-damaged skin by promoting collagen formation. This refreshing lotion will ease the pain of a sunburn and promote healing.

    ½ cup aloe vera gel
    ¼ cup carrot seed oil
    ¼ cup sesame oil
    1 tablespoon liquid vitamin E
    1 teaspoon liquid vitamin C
    5 drops lavender essential oil

Combine the aloe, carrot seed oil, and sesame oil in a blender. Buzz to blend. Add the vitamins E and C and the lavender essential oil, and process briefly. Pour into a clean container and cap tightly.

Body Powders

Body powders can wick away excess moisture and keep you cool and dry on the hottest day. But the powders we grew up with were often based on talc. For a healthier alternative, try one of these soothing formulas. Store your finished powder in a glass bottle with a shaker top or a jar large enough to accommodate a fluffy duster.

Silky French Lavender Bath Powder   Yield: 8 ounces
Step out of the shower and into a cloud of lavender-scented powder. This simple formula can also be adapted to use other herbal scents.

> 1 cup cornstarch
> ½ cup rice flour
> ¼ cup dried lavender flowers, finely crushed
> 4 drops lavender essential oil

Mix the ingredients in a glass bowl, stirring well to distribute the lavender and oil. Carefully pour the powder into a glass container with a shaker lid and cap tightly.

Deodorizing Powder   Yield: 12 ounces
Chase away body odor with baking soda and sage—two powerful odor eliminators. Unlike talc-based powders, this powder is safe to use on sanitary pads and undergarments. For best results, use after bathing or showering.

> ½ cup baking soda
> ½ cup cornstarch
> ½ cup arrowroot powder
> 8 drops sage essential oil

Combine the baking soda, cornstarch, and arrowroot in a glass bowl and stir well to mix. Add the essential oil, stirring again to disperse the oil throughout the mixture. Carefully pour the powder into a glass container with a shaker lid and cap tightly.

Warming Spice Bath Powder   YIELD: 8 ounces

This spice-scented powder is wonderfully warming after a hot bath on a cold winter night.

 1 cup cornstarch
 ½ teaspoon ground cinnamon
 ½ teaspoon ground cloves
 ½ teaspoon ground ginger
 ½ teaspoon ground nutmeg
 3 drops cinnamon essential oil

Combine the cinnamon, cloves, ginger, and nutmeg in a glass bowl and stir well to mix. Add the essential oil, stirring again to disperse the oil through-out the mixture. Carefully pour the powder into a glass container with a shaker lid and cap tightly.

Special Treatments

As the years pass, our bodies can become home to less-than-beautiful skin conditions. An aggressive game plan using these formulas can minimize these problems.

Body Blemish Gel   YIELD: 4 ounces

The pimples you thought you outgrew in your teens can suddenly appear on your body, thanks to excess perspiration or hormonal swings. This treatment uses lavender and tea tree oil—powerful antibacterial herbs that can help blemishes heal quickly.

 ½ cup aloe vera gel
 6 drops lavender essential oil
 6 drops tea tree oil

Combine the ingredients in a small glass bowl and whisk to blend thoroughly. Spoon into a container with a tight-fitting lid and store in the refrigerator.

Cellulite Cream   YIELD: 7 ounces

Combining this cream with skin brushing, exercise, and a healthy diet may help minimize the appearance of "orange-peel skin."

 1 tablespoon dulse
 1 tablespoon horsetail

 1 teaspoon ginger, freshly grated
 ½ cup distilled water
 2 ounces cocoa butter
 1 tablespoon beeswax, grated
 1 tablespoon wheat germ oil
 1 teaspoon liquid vitamin E
 1 teaspoon liquid vitamin C

Combine the dulse, horsetail, ginger, and water in a saucepan. Heat on high until boiling. Remove from heat and allow to steep for 20 minutes. Meanwhile, combine the cocoa butter, beeswax, and wheat germ oil in a glass bowl. Cover loosely and microwave on medium for 30 seconds. Stir and repeat, if necessary, until the cocoa butter and beeswax have melted completely.

Strain the herbal infusion, reserving the liquid. Slowly pour the liquid into the cocoa butter mixture, stirring constantly. Cool slightly and add the vitamins E and C. Pour the mixture into a clean glass jar and cool completely before capping. To use, massage a small amount into your skin where cellulite is present.

Stretch Mark Oil   YIELD: 12 ounces

As many pregnant women eventually discover, stretch marks are red or pink "scars" on the abdomen, hips, thighs, and breasts, which can develop during pregnancy. Although these scars eventually fade to white, most women would rather prevent, or at least minimize, these visible signs of motherhood.

 1 cup olive oil
 2 ounces cocoa butter
 1 tablespoon liquid vitamin E
 10 drops lavender essential oil

Combine the olive oil and cocoa butter in a small saucepan and heat gently until the cocoa butter has melted completely. Cool slightly before adding the vitamin E and essential oil. Pour into a glass bottle and cool completely before capping. To use, massage a generous amount into your skin.

This oil should be used daily from the third month of pregnancy and continued for six to eight weeks after delivery.

Shaving Aids

You may be surprised to find that regular shaving actually helps keep legs soft and smooth by gently exfoliating dead skin cells as you remove unwanted hair. Instead of shaving with chemical-filled shaving creams or drying soap and water, try these skin-pampering alternatives.

Silky Shaving Cream   Yield: 8 ounces

This soapless shaving cream soothes and moisturizes your skin as you shave, reducing the chance of razor burn.

> 1 cup aloe vera gel
> ½ teaspoon liquid vitamin E
> 5 drops chamomile essential oil
> 3 drops lavender essential oil
> 2 drops rose essential oil

Combine ingredients in a small glass bowl and mix with a wire whisk until thoroughly blended. Store in a plastic jar with a tight-fitting lid. To use, scoop up a handful of the gel and smooth it on your legs. Shave as usual. Rinse and pat dry with an absorbent towel.

After-Shave Mist   Yield: 12 ounces

Men have known for years that an after-shave lotion conditions the skin and closes the pores. Finally, here is a version specifically designed for women.

> ½ cup aloe vera gel
> ½ cup boiling distilled water
> ¼ cup calendula flowers
> ½ cup witch hazel
> 6 drops chamomile essential oil
> 3 drops lavender essential oil

Combine the aloe and water in a small saucepan. Bring to a boil. Meanwhile, tie the calendula into a cheesecloth square and secure with a string or rubber band. Place the packet into the boiling mixture and remove the pan from the heat. Allow to steep for 20 minutes.

Discard the packet and stir the witch hazel into the calendula infusion. Allow to cool completely. Add the chamomile and lavender essential oils, and stir to blend. Pour into a plastic spray bottle and cap tightly. To use, simply spray onto your freshly shaven skin.

Deodorants

It's not exactly a topic most folks like to talk about. After all, body odor isn't pleasant. Since perspiration-loving bacteria are the culprit behind the aroma, these deodorants are designed to keep bacteria in check.

Witchy Woman Deodorant Spray   YIELD: 8 ounces

This spray deodorant relies on bacteria-fighting herbs to prevent odor and on the antiseptic properties of witch hazel to discourage perspiration without clogging pores.

> ⅛ cup crushed coriander
> ½ cup fresh sage leaves
> ½ cup boiling distilled water
> ½ cup witch hazel
> ½ teaspoon liquid vitamin C
> 5 drops chamomile essential oil

Place the coriander and sage in a small bowl, and pour the boiling water over the herbs. Allow to steep for 20 minutes. Strain into a clean plastic container or spray bottle. Add the witch hazel, vitamin C, and essential oil. Cap tightly and shake to mix. To use, either spray under your arms or apply with a cotton ball.

Rose Antiperspirant Spray   YIELD: 8 ounces

Rose water is a natural astringent that can help reduce perspiration. It also has the reputation for soothing irritated skin, making it ideal for use on tender underarms.

> ½ cup rose water
> ½ cup witch hazel
> 3 drops chamomile essential oil

Combine the ingredients in a spray bottle. Shake well to mix.

Sage Cream Deodorant   YIELD: 5 ounces

Some women prefer a cream deodorant, particularly if they have dry skin. This formula uses sage for its deodorizing properties.

> ¼ cup almond oil
> 1 tablespoon avocado oil

2 teaspoons beeswax, grated

8 drops sage essential oil

3 drops grapefruit seed extract

Combine the almond oil, avocado oil, and beeswax in a small saucepan. Heat gently until the beeswax has melted completely. Cool. Stir in the essential oil and extract and spoon into a clean jar with a tight-fitting lid. To use, massage a small amount under arms.

❧ Smart Shopping ☙

Can you pamper your body with off-the-shelf bath and body products and still avoid chemical cocktails? Of course! Whether you are bathing, exfoliating, soothing, smoothing, or deodorizing, these natural products can provide a healthy alternative. Just remember to check the list of ingredients on the label since some natural products do contain preservatives.

Bath Oils

Manufacturer	Product
Aubrey Organics	Blue Camomile Bath Oil
Burt's Bees	Vitamin E Body and Bath Oil
EO	Bath Soaks
Essential Elements	Aromatherapy Bath Beads

Bath Salts

Manufacturer	Product
Abra Therapeutics	Cellular Detox Bath
	Cold and Flu Bath
	Energy Tonic Bath
	Menopause Bath
	Moisture Therapy Bath
	Muscle Therapy Bath

	PMS Therapy Bath
	Sleep Therapy Bath
	Stress Therapy Bath
Ancient Secrets	Aromatherapy Dead Sea Mineral Salts
Aura Cacia	Mineral Baths
Beeswork	Chamomile Bath Salts
	EuroSpice Bath Salts
	Lavender Bath Salts
Better Botanicals	Dead Sea Bath Salts
Burt's Bees	Bath Salts
	Buttermilk Bath
	Green Goddess Bath Salts
	Green Goddess Emollient Milk Bath
	Green Goddess Juniper and Cypress Bath
	Ocean Potion Dead Sea Salts
	Ocean Potion Detox Dulse Bath
	Therapeutic Bath Crystals
Dr. Hauschka	Lavender Bath
	Lemon Bath
	Rosemary Bath
	Sage Bath
	Spruce Bath
EO	Bath Salts
Essential Elements	Citrus Dream Bath Salts
	Fleur D'Amour Bath Salts
	Joie De Lavender Bath Salts
	Wake Up Rosemary Bath Salts
Masada	Mineral Herb Spa
NaturElle	Energizing Mineral Bath
	Purifying Mineral Bath
	Relaxing Mineral Bath

Bubble Baths

Manufacturer	*Product*
Aubrey Organics	Camomile Bubbles Herbal Bath Oil
Neways	Indulge Bubble Bath

Body Cleansers

Manufacturer	Product
Aubrey Organics	Herbal Liquid Body Soap
	Rosa Mosqueta Rose Hip Liquid Soap
Avalon	Liquid Soap
Better Botanicals	Botanical Body Wash
Compliments of Nature	Organic Herbal Body Wash
Dr. Hauschka	Holistic Body Wash Floral
Jakaré	Moisturizing Body Wash
Perfectly Beautiful	Radiant Skin Hand and Body Cleanser
Sun Dog	Hemp Oil Liquid Soap

Shower Gels

Manufacturer	Product
Avalon	Therapeutic Bath and Shower Gel
EO	ShowerGel
Essential Elements	Citrus Dream Shower Gel
	Wake Up Rosemary Shower Gel
NaturElle	Head-To-Toe All-Over Wash
	Invigorating Bath and Shower Gel
	Super-Gentle Shower and Bath Gel

Exfoliators/Body Scrubs

Manufacturer	Product
Compliments of Nature	Chocolate Mint Body Scrub
Trillium Herbal Co.	Organic Body Polish

Body Lotions

Manufacturer	Product
Aubrey Organics	Blue Green Algae Hand and Body Lotion
	Evening Primrose Lotion
Beeswork	Nature's Lotion
Better Botanicals	Botanical Body Blend
	Kokum Butter Body Balm

Botanics of California	Grapefruit Body Lotion
Burt's Bees	Carrot Nutrition
	Milk and Honey Body Lotion
Dr. Hauschka	Body Milk
	Rose Body Milk
	Rosemary Leg and Arm Toner
Essential Elements	Citrus Dream Hand and Body Lotion
	Fleur D'Amour Hand and Body Lotion
	Joie De Lavender Hand and Body Lotion
	Wake Up Rosemary Hand and Body Lotion
NaturElle	Green Tea Anti-Oxidant Moisturizing Body Lotion
Neways	Tender Care
Paul Penders	Carotene Head-To-Toe
Penny Island	Pure Rose Geranium Hand and Body Lotion
	Real Vanilla and Lavender Hand/Body Lotion
	Simply Fragrance Free Hand and Body Lotion
	Sweet Almond Hand and Body Lotion
Real Purity	Extra Rich Hand and Body Lotion
Rich's	MSM Non-Fragrance Lotion

Body Powders

Manufacturer	Product
Dr. Hauschka	Body Powder
EO	Body Powders

Cellulite Creams

Manufacturer	Product
Burt's Bees	Ocean Potion Cellulite Creme

Shaving Aids

Manufacturer	Product
Beeswork	Nature's Shave
Desert Essence	Shaving Oil
Paul Penders	Silky Smooth Shave Cream
Real Purity	Shave Creme

Waxes/Sugaring Compounds

Manufacturer	Product
Moom	Sugaring Compound
Touchme	Sugaring Gel

Deodorants

Manufacturer	Product
Aubrey Organics	Calendula Blossom Natural Deodorant Spray
	E Plus High C Roll-On Deodorant
Avalon	Therapeutic Deodorant
Burt's Bees	Herbal Deodorant
Dr. Hauschka	Deodorant, Floral Scent
	Deodorant, Fresh Scent
Earth Science	Tea Tree Oil Natural Herbal Deodorant
Home Health	Roll-On Deodorant
Neways	Subdue Deodorant
Real Purity	Deodorant
Weleda	Citrus Deodorant
	Sage Deodorant

Antiperspirants

Manufacturer	Product
Crystal	Stick Deodorant
The Natural	Stick Deodorant
Natural Crystal	Deodorant Spray with Aloe Vera
	Stick Deodorant

8

Scentual Magic: Fragrances

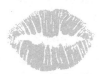

"Of all the senses, none surely is so mysterious as that of smell."
—Dr. D. McKenzie, *Study of Smells*

The soothing scent of lavender, the comforting fragrance of freshly baked bread, the invigorating aroma of newly cut grass. Experiencing a favorite scent not only brings us sensory pleasure but also can stir our emotions or evoke fond memories of people, places, and events that have played a significant role in our lives. Our sense of smell envelops life's aromas, letting us savor the nuances and chords of each scent.

The human nose can distinguish among thousands of unique odors, thanks to approximately one thousand specialized sensory receptors. When a receptor encounters an odor, it sends a signal to the olfactory bulb, a brain structure just above the nose. From there, the information is relayed to other parts of the brain. Can scent really influence how we feel? In a study by the University of Vienna, Austria, when subjects were exposed to 1,8-cineol, a stimulating synthetic fragrance, measurable responses could be seen in the cerebral blood flow.[1] Researchers hope that by learning more about the olfactory/brain connection, they will eventually understand the exact chemical and biological interactions that give fragrance the power to affect our thoughts, emotions, and behavior.

From Sheba to Synthetics

Fragrance has always held a special place in society. Throughout history, humans have used various scents for everything from religious rituals to aphrodisiacs. The Egyptians were the first to integrate perfume into their culture in the form of incense. In fact, the word *perfume* comes from the Latin *per fume*, or "through smoke," a term that reflects this early use of scent.

It wasn't long before scented balms and ointments were created by the high priests, who used fragrance to carry out their religious, medicinal, and embalming duties. But fragrance didn't remain within the bounds of the religious world. Led by the Queen of Sheba, Egyptians soon discovered the cosmetic value of scent. To meet the demand, the very same priests who created fragrances for their religious rites became the first manufacturers of perfume for the rich and powerful classes. Encased in beautiful and expensive alabaster, onyx, or blown glass containers, fragrant extracts of rose, henna, lily, cinnamon, and peppermint made their way into the baths and boudoirs of well-to-do people. As trade routes expanded, so did the use of perfume. Although each corner of the world used scent in slightly different ways, the common thread was that all perfume was based in nature.

The development of organic chemistry in the late nineteenth century changed the very essence of how perfume was created and used. Suddenly, synthetic perfume materials could be developed in a laboratory. Generally less expensive than their natural counterparts, synthetic fragrance ingredients could be created year-round, solving the problem of seasonal availability. The invention of gas chromatography and mass spectrometry enabled chemists to analyze natural materials and duplicate the various components contained in a single plant. By adding these synthetics to natural ingredients, perfumers could develop thousands of different fragrances. Instead of the harmonious blending designed by nature, perfume manufacturers could now use a variety of unrelated components assembled at random to achieve a marketable product.

Scent Sells

Fragrance is big business—so big that it represents 45 percent of all cosmetics dollars spent in the United States.[2] In 1997 alone, the fragrance industry realized profits of more than $5 billion.[3] Driving these profits are skillfully created marketing campaigns that convince consumers that the proper scent can make them feel fresh, confident, and alluring.

It all begins with the product's name. What's in a name? When it comes to fragrance, everything! A perfume's name can convey a specific "feeling" to the consumer. Calvin Klein's "Obsession" is designed to give users the illusion of forbidden passion. Coty's "Adidas Moves for Her" creates the aura of athletic performance. Estée Lauder's "Honeysuckle Splash" evokes youth and innocence. Creating the proper name can make or break the success of a perfume. With the right name for a product, advertisers can create an entire fantasy designed to lure consumers to their particular scent. These mega-media campaigns don't come cheap. It's not unusual for a manufacturer to spend $3 million to $4 million to launch a new fragrance in hopes of realizing profits of $25 million or more.[4]

How the product is packaged is another important selling point. The shape and color of a bottle of perfume can further enhance the illusion by appealing to our senses of touch and sight. Angular lines can signal bold confidence, elegant cut glass stirs our feminine side, and soft, flowing curves spark images of sensuality. Although perfume bottles can be an art form in themselves, what's in those beautifully chiseled bottles may not be quite so alluring.

Eau de Chemical

Secrecy and intrigue have always been a part of the fragrance industry. Since fragrances can't be patented, formulas have historically been a closely guarded secret within this highly competitive business. This shroud of secrecy was designed to protect against imitators looking to steal a perfumer's trade secrets. Because of this cloak-and-dagger mentality, fragrance products, unlike cosmetics, have never been required to list their ingredients, making it all but impossible for consumers to know what they are really buying.

It's estimated that there are between three thousand and five thousand fragrance ingredients available to modern perfumers. Of these, it's believed that 95 percent are created in the laboratory, many from petroleum products. While this gives manufacturers the advantage of using numerous components not found in nature, 84 percent of the ingredients contained in synthetic fragrances have never been tested for safety.

In 1986, the National Academy of Sciences targeted six categories of chemicals that should be tested for neurotoxicity. Among them were insecticides, heavy metals, solvents, and fragrances. In its report, presented to the U.S. House of Representatives Committee on Science and Technology, it noted that petroleum-based ingredients, including benzene derivatives and alde-hydes commonly found in fragrance, were capable of causing cancer, birth defects, central nervous system disorders, and allergic reactions.[5]

So, what's really lurking in that beautiful bottle of perfume? When you purchase one of the mass-marketed perfumes, you may be getting anywhere from ten to three hundred ingredients in a single bottle. Although modern-day perfumes still contain some natural elements that would be familiar to our ancestors, most of the ingredients are synthetically created. Essential oils and resins can now be synthesized to mimic nature at a small fraction of the cost. For example, a kilogram of pure rose oil would cost a perfume manu-facturer $5,000. By using rose oil's chief constituent, phenyl ethyl alcohol, a synthetic version of the same scent can be made for only $10 a kilogram.[6] While these synthetic ingredients have made fragrance affordable to all women, what is the long-term cost to their health?

In 1991, the Environmental Protection Agency (EPA) tested thirty-one fragrance products, including soaps, deodorants, hair sprays, perfumes, and colognes.[7] The intent of the study was to identify the toxicological properties of various fragrances that pose a risk to human health and contribute to indoor air pollution. One of the products tested was a popular designer per-fume, which was found to contain:

beta-pinene	camphene
benzaldehyde	2-ethyl-1-hexanol
benzyl alcohol	3,7-dimethyl-1,3,7-octatriene
linalool	$C_{15}H_{24}$
benzyl acetate	crotonaldehyde
alpha-terpineol	2-furaldehyde
beta-citronellol	gamma-terpinolene
ethanol	alpha-terpinolene
limonene	phenyl acetaldehyde
beta-phenethyl alcohol	o-allytoluene
beta-myrcene	acetophenone
alpha-cedrene	allocimene
t-butanol	2-methyl-4-phenyl-1-butene
ethyl acetate	carvone
toluene	

Although the EPA was able to pinpoint certain toxic substances in the products tested, the researchers confronted an alarming lack of information for many of the compounds investigated. The extant information suggested that these chemicals have a relatively low toxicity. However, the researchers did note positive results for toxic effects of some compounds previously thought benign, even at low doses. Many of the ingredients in this particular perfume are also named under the EPA's Toxic Substance Control Act, including allocimene, benzyl acetate, camphene, carvone, ethyl acetate, 2-ethyl-1-hexanol, 2-furaldehyde, limonene, and linalool.

Technical information culled from the Material Safety Data Sheets shows that the toxicological properties for some of the twenty-nine chemicals listed have not been thoroughly investigated.[8] Nevertheless, enough is known about these particular chemicals to raise red flags among researchers, manufacturers, and government regulators. For instance, many are skin and/or respiratory irritants, including allocimene, alpha-cedrene, alpha-terpineol, beta-citronellol, beta-myrcene, beta-pinene, camphene, carvone, 2-ethyl-1-hexanol, limonene, and linalool.[9]

Worse yet, some ingredients in this high-priced fragrance can affect the reproductive or central nervous system. Benzaldehyde, ethyl acetate, and t-butanol, for instance, have a narcotic effect that depresses the central nervous system. T-butanol and toluene can affect a developing fetus. Some of these same chemicals are also listed as possible carcinogens by the State of California, the National Toxicology Program, or the EPA, including benzaldehyde, benzyl alcohol, benzyl acetate, 2-furaldehyde, and acetophenone.[10]

Unfortunately, this specific product isn't the exception when it comes to synthetic perfumes and colognes. It's the rule. Department and drugstore scents are full of chemicals that may have an adverse effect on your health and the health of those around you.

Death by Perfume

While it may sound like something out of an Agatha Christie novel, for anyone sensitive to the chemicals in perfume, associating death with synthetic fragrance may be closer to fact than fiction. After being attacked by a patient who sprayed perfume in her face, one twenty-one-year-old medical assistant thought she was suffocating. She felt her throat and face swell up and experienced shortness of breath before collapsing to the floor. This acute anaphylactic reaction has left her with persistent shortness of breath and an intolerance to all perfumes months after the incident.[11]

Although such violent reactions have always been considered a rarity, they are becoming more common. For example, Denel, a mother of seven, didn't even know she was chemically sensitive until an exposure while she was pregnant triggered a severe reaction. Now each exposure can bring on migraine-like headaches and gastrointestinal problems. "After I'm around someone wearing perfume, I'll throw up all night," Denel says. "The worst experience was when I was stuck in an elevator with someone drenched in cologne. I was sick for days."

While Denel has never been able to identify which particular chemical triggers this violent response, Myrna, a retired teacher and artist, knows exactly what her problem is. "It's the formaldehyde," Myrna explains. "Whenever I come in contact with anyone wearing a fragrance containing formaldehyde, I become disoriented and suffer short-term memory loss. It's as if my brain is enveloped in a fog." A severe exposure can also leave Myrna with breathing problems and muscle weakness. Exposed to pesticides as a child, Myrna suffers from asthma and a weakened immune system. She cites this early environmental assault as the cause of the chemical sensitivity she experiences today.

These three women exemplify the growing number of people who suffer from fragrance-related chemical sensitivity. Some authorities estimate that 15 percent or more of the general population is plagued by some form of chemical sensitivity.[12] The symptoms can be as mild as a few sneezes or as debilitating as migraines, upper respiratory problems, and neurological disturbances. Unfortunately, this growing problem has historically been dismissed by the fragrance industry, government regulators, and the medical community. Women who seek treatment for fragrance-related health problems have often been told that "it's all in your head."

One reason doctors have such a difficult time diagnosing chemical sensitivities is that the physical manifestation of a sensitivity is often a result of cumulative exposure. Fragrances that seem to be well tolerated for years can suddenly cause problems, making it hard to pinpoint the exact cause. Since the cause is often elusive, many primary care physicians deny the existence of fragrance-induced illness, instead urging chemically sensitive patients to seek psychological counseling. Yet, it is a real health problem for those suffering from fragrance-related sensitivities. Even casual exposure to another's fragrance can bring on symptoms of dizziness; nausea; muscle weakness; loss of concentration; and eye, throat, and lung irritation. Many people with acute sensitivities have been forced into a hermitlike existence. The widespread use of fragrance has created a barrier that prevents people with chemical sensitivities from participating in work or social activities. Even simple tasks such as grocery shopping can become a triggering event. In a world where fragrance is in everything from perfume to laundry detergent to toilet paper, it's nearly impossible to find a fragrance-free oasis. People with chemical sensitivities have had to protect their health the only way they know how—by withdrawing from life itself.

Fortunately, several studies give credibility to people who are intolerant to fragrance. An animal study conducted by Vermont-based Anderson Laboratories found that some fragrance products emit chemicals that cause a variety of acute toxicities in mice. The authors of the study observed: "The emissions of these fragrance products caused various combinations of sensory irritation, pulmonary irritation, decreases in expiratory airflow velocity, as well as alterations of the functional observational battery indicative of neurotoxicity. Neurotoxicity was more severe after mice were repeatedly exposed."[13] Also, a study by researchers in Lexington, Virginia, found evidence that even low-level exposure can result in behavioral and cognitive effects.[14]

Exposure to the chemicals in perfumes and colognes may also be a contributing factor in the skyrocketing number of asthma cases that have been diagnosed over the past two decades. According to the American Lung Association, asthma affects more than 17.7 million Americans and kills more than five thousand each year.[15] Although exposure to air pollution, dust, and pet dander can trigger an asthma attack, the most frequent offender is fragrance. One small Swedish study discovered that perfume can provoke an asthma attack and respiratory problems even when subjects are prevented from smelling the perfume.[16] A study by Louisiana State University found that the scented perfume strips that commonly litter women's magazines caused airway obstruction, chest tightness, and wheezing in asthmatics.[17] And Tulane University Medical Center conducted a study that identified thirty-eight brand-name fragrances that prompted a decline in lung function. Of those, the top six offenders were Red, White Diamonds, Giorgio, Charlie, Opium, and Poison.[18]

Adverse reactions to perfume can manifest themselves in other ways too. According to the American Academy of Dermatology, fragrances cause more allergic contact dermatitis than any other cosmetic ingredient and may affect nearly 10 percent of the population.[19] An allergic reaction can show itself immediately or can crop up seven to ten days after the first exposure. Symptoms can include redness, swelling, rashes, hives, or, in severe cases, eczema and are usually located on the face, eyelids, neck, and hands. Although the problem usually disappears after a week or so, once a reaction has occurred, any contact with the allergen will cause a relapse.

Migraines can also be triggered by exposure to fragrance.[20] Migraines are a serious and debilitating disease that affects between 11 million and 18 million Americans, most of them women.[21] It's believed that migraines are caused by a dilation of the blood vessels in the brain; the result can be intense pain, visual disturbances, and nausea. Scientists have found that some of the chemicals in fragrance have a direct effect on the brain, altering the flow of blood,[22] and believe there may be a link between fragrance and migraines. Even low-level or undetected odors may be triggers.[23]

Switching to unscented products may not protect you from chemical sensitivities or an allergic reaction. An investigation by Boston's New England Medical Center Hospital found that even products that promote themselves as "fragance-free" may contain raw fragrance ingredients.[24] According to the Food and Drug Administration (FDA), the terms *fragrance-free* and *unscented* have no legal definition.[25] While these terms imply that the product has no perceptible odor, manufacturers do add masking fragrances to hide unpleasant odors.

Although the acute reactions discussed so far can be disruptive, even debilitating, the long-term impact of fragrance chemicals can be deadly. Many of the chemicals commonly included in perfume are listed as potentially carcinogenic to the liver and kidneys, including acetophenone, benzaldehyde, benzyl acetate, and 2-furaldehyde. Terpineol, which is also widely used in perfume, was found to be mutagenic by Brazilian researchers.[26] And a National Institute of Occupational Safety and Health animal study found that benzoin, another common ingredient in fragrance, caused enlarged lymph nodes in both male and female mice and enlarged spleens in males. The study also cited benzoin's potential to cause liver damage.[27]

Since perfume can enter the body either through the skin or by inhalation, many of the toxins in perfumes and colognes are readily absorbed. Some of these, particularly synthetic musks, have been shown to accumulate in the body's fatty tissues and have been detected in human breast milk.[28] One synthetic musk, musk xylene, was detected in the blood of both animal and human subjects.[29] Other fragrance chemicals are reproductive toxicants. Animal studies of glycol esters have shown that even low-dose exposures can increase the risk of infertility, spontaneous abortion, and birth defects.[30] And toluene and t-butanol are both fetotoxic.[31] These hormone disruptors can silently accumulate within the human body over many years, with potentially devastating effects.

Scented Seafood?

These endocrine-disrupting fragrance chemicals can also impact the environment. Until recently, the bioactive chemicals in fragrance received little attention as potential environmental pollutants. But when traces of synthetic musks began showing up in fish, researchers suddenly began to take notice.[32]

Musks are considered an essential ingredient in perfumes because of their musky scent and their ability to make a fragrance last longer. Older synthetic musks, such as musk ketone and musk xylene, and the newer polycyclic musk fragrances, hexahydro-hexamethylcyclopental-benzopyran (HHCB) and acetylhexamethyltetralin (AHTN), have also turned up in water, sewage sludge, and aquatic species around the world.[33] Potentially more dangerous are the by-products produced as these synthetic musks degrade.[34] Studies of musk compounds in sewage sludge have documented that, as the chemicals break down, their by-products are found in higher concentrations.[35]

Synthetic musks are persistent environmental pollutants that can accumulate in the fatty tissue of wildlife. Fish and other aquatic life-forms exposed to low levels can suffer subtle biological changes over the course of several generations. Although the environmental impact of these changes is not known, what is known is that these pollutants eventually make their way into the human food chain. Although no one can predict the long-term health effects of eating contaminated fish, drinking musk-laced water, and using fragrances containing synthetic musks, Dr. Christian Daughton, a researcher with the Environmental Sciences Division of the EPA's National Exposure Research Laboratory, has noted that the human concentration of musk—the amount stored in a person's fatty tissue—is similar to that of PCBs.[36]

Fragrance chemicals also affect the air we breathe. The volatile compounds in perfumes contribute to indoor air pollution. An analysis of perfume by Scientific Instrument Services, a New Jersey supplier of mass spectrometers, gas chromatographs, and liquid chromatographs, identified more than eight hundred compounds from six perfumes that may contribute to indoor air pollution.[37] Among them were acetone, benzaldehyde, benzyl alcohol, diethyl phthalate, and musk ketone. More frightening, studies have documented that fragrance-related air pollution isn't confined to indoor spaces. Researchers have detected both polycyclic and nitro musks in Norwegian outdoor air samples.[38] Concentrations ranged from low levels to hundreds of picograms per cubic meter. While the amount may sound small, the health implications of breathing in these contaminants on a continual basis may prove to be a much larger health issue.

Who's Minding the Industry?

In light of the mounting evidence that many fragrance chemicals pose health and environmental risks, you may wonder why nothing has been done to rein in the fragrance industry's use of these toxic compounds. While government regulation for cosmetics is, at best, limited and outdated, government oversight for fragrances is virtually nonexistent. Even though perfumes and other scented products fall under the jurisdiction of the FDA, the fragrance industry is essentially self-regulated. Because of the long-standing tradition of trade secrets, ingredient labels are not compulsory, and no preapproval safety testing is required for the raw fragrance materials used.[39]

So, who is watching over the industry? That responsibility falls to the Research Institute for Fragrance Materials (RIFM), an industry-sponsored nonprofit organization charged with evaluating the safety of fragrance ingredients. Established in 1966 after a wave of consumer complaints regarding fragrance-related skin reactions and threats of regulation, the RIFM tests only raw fragrance materials selected by its Scientific Advisory Board, whose members are from the industry itself.[40] According to Richard Ford, former vice president of the organization, "Over the approximately thirty years since its inception, RIFM has tested virtually all important fragrance material in common use."[41] Yet, only thirteen hundred of the more than five thousand chemicals used in perfume have been evaluated.[42] Moreover, the testing that is done is limited to acute oral and dermal toxicity, dermal irritation and sensitization, and phototoxicity evaluations. The respiratory or neurotoxic effects of these chemicals are not investigated, nor are the chemicals tested for their potential as carcinogens or endocrine disruptors.

Once the RIFM has completed the testing process, the results are sent to the International Fragrance Association (IFRA), an organization made up of more than one hundred fragrance manufacturers representing fifteen countries. Based on the information from the RIFM, the IFRA compiles and publishes safety recommendations for use by the industry. This "Code of Practice" currently recommends against the use of more than thirty fragrance compounds and advises limiting the use of many more. However, the IFRA has no authority to enforce the guidelines, and no one monitors products to see that they are being followed.

Even though the RIFM tests for common allergens, it's estimated that 50 percent of all cosmetics allergies are fragrance related. That figure is rapidly rising as dermatologists are treating an ever-increasing number of patients with fragrance dermatitis. In response, the American Academy of Dermatology has urged fragrance trade associations and manufacturers to adopt voluntary ingredient labeling for all cosmetic products containing fragrance.[43] So far, no one in the fragrance industry is paying much attention.

Although the industry insists that current safety-testing measures are adequate, past performance raises some questions. In 1975, routine irritancy tests of acetyl ethyl tetramethyl tetralin (AETT), a synthetic nitro musk used widely in perfumes, colognes, and other fragrance products, uncovered some disturbing results. The researchers observed that the rats used in the experiments developed an extraordinary blue discoloration of their skin and internal organs. What's more, the animals began to display unusual behavior, and it was discovered that the insulating sheath surrounding the nerves that connect the brain cells was degenerating. Further research at the Albert Einstein College of Medicine in the Bronx, New York, confirmed that AETT did indeed cause serious brain damage in animals.[44] When news of these findings became known, the fragrance industry voluntarily discontinued use of AETT— twenty-two years after the chemical began appearing in consumer products. It took another three years before this voluntary industry action was acknowledged by the FDA.

Another synthetic musk, 2,6-dinitro-3-methoxy-4-tert-butyltoluene, more commonly known as musk ambrette, was also found to be a neurotoxin. This chemical has been used since the 1920s as a fragrance fixative. Studies in 1967 found that mice that had been fed musk ambrette developed limb weakness and other neurotoxic symptoms. In addition, musk ambrette was discovered to be phototoxic. But because dietary exposure to this chemical is extremely low, the research was discounted. Then in 1985, another animal study showed that musk ambrette damages the central nervous system when applied to the skin.[45] This time the IFRA listened and recommended that perfumers refrain from using musk ambrette in their formulations. However, to this day, the FDA simply lists musk ambrette as a photocontact sensitizer.[46]

An ocean away, the European Commission is taking action to protect consumers from the adverse effects of fragrance. Premarketing notifications are now required under the European Directive on Dangerous Substances. The new law states that, before any new chemical can be introduced, specific testing and reporting must be done to determine its health and environmental impact. Since testing just one compound can be an expensive undertaking, fragrance manufacturers are understandably unhappy about the new European requirements.[47]

The Politics of Scent

The current system of self-regulation may work for the fragrance industry and government regulators, but it doesn't sit well with consumer groups. One California group, the Environmental Health Network (EHN), recently filed a petition with the FDA to have Calvin Klein's fragrance Eternity declared misbranded. The basis for the petition was an independent analysis commissioned by the EHN that revealed that the popular scent contained forty-one chemicals, including diethyl phthalate, a suspected hormone disruptor; hydrocinnamaldehyde, which targets the male reproductive organs; phenols, a suspected carcinogen that may cause reproductive damage; benzenethanol, a neurotoxin; synthetic musks; and a variety of skin and respiratory irritants.[48] Endorsing the EHN's efforts is the Cancer Prevention Coalition, a nationwide coalition of cancer prevention and public health experts; citizen activists; and labor, environmental, and women's health groups.[49]

The San Francisco and Loma Prieta chapters of the Sierra Club have also resolved to "take action to discourage the use of fragrance products in all public places." It's a position they would like to become a national policy.[50] Limiting the use of fragrance may be an idea whose time has come. Fragrance-free zones are gaining attention across the country. One federal agency, the U.S. Architectural and Transportation Barriers Compliance Board, has even voted to adopt a fragrance-free policy and has notified the public that "persons attending board meetings are requested to refrain from using perfume, cologne, and other fragrances for the comfort of other participants."[51]

A growing number of communities are also opting for a reduction in secondhand fragrance. Halifax, Nova Scotia, has established fragrance-free policies in its public buildings. Taking the city's lead, many private businesses have followed suit. Scents are also getting the thumbs-down in some social settings. The Seattle Folklore Society has adopted a fragrance-free policy for its English country dances.[52] And the hungry citizens of Marin County, California, are now able to choose a fragrance-free table at their favorite restaurant.[53]

Good Scents

Some manufacturers are paying attention to consumer health concerns. Over the past decade, natural perfumes and colognes have begun popping up in health food stores and natural salons for those who want to enjoy fragrance without the chemical consequences. These simple scents are based on natural alcohol and essential oils. Scented waters are another nontoxic alternative. Although *any* scent can trigger an adverse reaction in chemically sensitive individuals, using these natural scents is a much safer way to add fragrance to your life.

Essential oils have been used safely for thousands of years as a basis for perfume. Unlike synthetic perfume or fragrance oils, which are isolates of a single plant molecule, essential oils contain a harmonious blend of natural constituents. Highly concentrated, pure essential oils are created through the process of either steam distillation or expression.

Steam distillation extracts the essential oil through condensation. As the plant oils mix with the steam, they are carried up to a condenser, where the steam and oils separate. As the steam returns to its water state, the oil rises to the surface, where it can be easily collected. Expression, on the other hand, is a technique that presses the oils from the plant material; traditionally, the oils were then collected with sponges. Originally done by hand, expression can now be accomplished mechanically. Both techniques are time-consuming and yield minute amounts of oil—one reason pure essential oils are more expensive than other fragrance ingredients. Another reason is that huge quantities of plant material are required to produce small amounts of essential oil. For example, 440 pounds of lavender are needed to make 2.5 pounds of essential oil.[54] And just 1 pound of rose essential oil requires 5,000 pounds of rose petals.[55]

Some manufacturers have discovered a more economical technique to coerce the oils from botanicals. Volatile solvents are used to extract the oils from the plants. When the chemical solvent evaporates, a concentrated residue of the oil remains. Benzene, a solvent derived from coal tar, was the original solvent of choice. However, it fell out of favor because of the chemical's toxic effect on bone marrow and its ability to irritate the skin and mucous membranes.[56] Hexane, another petroleum solvent, eventually replaced the benzene traditionally used to extract oils. Consumers should be aware that essential oils extracted by this method contain trace amounts of the solvent used and cannot be considered pure essential oils.

A new method of obtaining a plant's essential oils, hypercritical carbon dioxide extraction, replaces the volatile solvents with liquid CO_2. Proponents say that this method offers the advantage of capturing volatile plant compounds not extracted under normal steam distillation. They also claim that the CO_2 is completely removed just by releasing the pressure in the extraction chamber, leaving no residue behind.[57] Critics, on the other hand, charge that CO_2 extraction will give the essential oils unfamiliar characteristics, virtually creating a new product whose safety and therapeutic qualities are not known.[58] But according to aromatherapist Christoph Streicher, Ph.D., president of Amrita Aromatherapy, essential oils derived by CO_2 extraction are just as pure as their steam-distilled counterparts. And, notes Streicher, this method is particularly effective for extracting the volatile compounds from dried plants and seeds.

Although you can buy an over-the-counter natural perfume, many women are beginning to purchase pure essential oils to create their own fragrance products. But be forewarned: essential oils aren't for everyone. Some botanicals can aggravate chemical sensitivities and may cause allergy and photosensitivity. If you can tolerate essential oils, let the following guidelines govern your purchases:

- **Quality costs.** When it comes to essential oils, you usually get what you pay for.
- **Beware of imposters.** The label should list the product as a *pure* essential oil. Avoid products labeled as essence oils, perfume oils, or fragrance oils.
- **Look for color variations.** Pure essential oils vary in color. For example, patchouli and thyme have a dark color, lavender has a light golden hue, and rosemary produces a clear essential oil. Products that are uniform in color, regardless of their scent, are usually synthetic.

• **Look for a warning label.** Essential oils should never be used "neat." A label that states that the product is concentrated or should not be used undiluted on the skin is an indication that you are buying a pure essential oil.

Some essential oils are diluted in a carrier oil such as jojoba or almond oil, a fact that will be stated on the label. The reason for the dilution is that some plant oils are extremely expensive to produce. Rose, neroli, and jasmine are among the more common essential oils diluted in a carrier. While this formulation may not be acceptable for therapeutic uses, a good-quality blend of pure oils is perfectly acceptable for making perfume.

Creating your own simple perfumes and colognes from essential oils is a relatively easy art to learn. With a little practice, you will begin to understand the basic fragrance properties of each oil and how to harmoniously blend them to create a unique scent all your own.

Essential oils also have medicinal or therapeutic properties that should be taken into account when blending perfumes. Aromatherapy, the science of using essential oils to enhance wellness, has gained enormous popularity in recent years. Alternative and conventional health practitioners have discovered its benefits for a variety of ailments. In fact, studies have shown that aromatherapy does produce physiological and psychological benefits.[59] Researchers have actually measured the effects of certain essential oils on mood, brain waves, and nerve impulses,[60] and aromatherapy has been found to be effective in the treatment of chronic pain, psoriasis, and alopecia areata, an autoimmune disease that results in hair loss.[61]

Although aromatherapy has a long and well-respected history of use, the fragrance industry might have dealt a blow to this healing art. Because of the growing popularity of this alternative therapy, cosmetics companies are now offering artificially scented products under the guise of aromatherapy. These products are usually packed with synthetic chemicals and contain perhaps a tiny smattering of essential oils. Be aware that the term *aromatherapy*, like the words *natural* and *botanical*, means absolutely nothing in the world of conventional cosmetics. It is simply a marketing tool designed to sell more product.

The oils listed in Table 8.1 should *not* be used for any kind of skin application, including perfumes and colognes.

Table 8.1 ❧ Hazardous Essential Oils

Angelica Root	phototoxic
Cassia	a powerful skin irritant and sensitizer
Cinnamon	a skin sensitizer at all concentrations
Pennyroyal	toxic
Peru Balsam	a skin sensitizer
Rue	a powerful photosensitizer and irritant
Sassafras	a possible carcinogen
Tansy	extremely toxic
Tolu Balsam	a skin sensitizer
Verbena	a powerful skin sensitizer and irritant
Wintergreen	may cause toxicity
Wormseed	extremely toxic

The Art of Perfume

Long before the age of synthetics, making perfume was an art. Perfumers would combine the essence of flowers and plant resins to create a harmonious blend of aromas, much like a beautiful piece of music. Like a composer, perfumers would expertly fashion a symphony of fragrant notes that would swell and fade over the course of a few hours. The "top notes" of a perfume, often referred to as the head, are the most volatile and evaporate quickly. The "middle notes" are the essence of the fragrance and are known as the heart of the perfume. Finally, the "base notes" add depth and longevity to the scent. Although each note has an aroma all its own, when it's blended with the other notes, a fragrant emotion is created.

Blending essential oils to create a pleasing effect requires as much intuition as practice. Beginning home perfumers should start with a simple blend containing no more than three essential oils. Choose a top, middle, and base note. A good ratio is 3:2:1. Since all essential oils possess antibacterial properties, it isn't necessary to add a natural preservative unless you are using a carrier oil that spoils rapidly. Vitamin E is a natural preservative that won't interfere with the scent you are creating. Simply add a quarter teaspoon of liquid vitamin E to your blend before mixing.

Many formulas for simple perfumes and colognes call for some sort of alcohol, usually vodka, to dilute the essential oils. But vodka has its drawbacks. First, you must cure the scent for four to six weeks to allow the alcohol and oils to blend—and to avoid smelling like a cocktail. Vodka also causes the mixture to separate into layers during the curing process since it does not contain enough alcohol to thoroughly dissolve the oils. Finally, any type of alcohol evaporates quickly, making it necessary to reapply your perfume every hour or two. It is better to dilute your essential oil blend in a good-quality carrier oil. Not only will you be able to wear the fragrance immediately, but also, the scent will last much longer than an alcohol-based perfume. Good carrier oils include avocado, grape seed, jojoba, and sunflower oils. Light colognes and toilet waters can be made by using essential oils diluted in distilled water. After you've made your fragrance, store it in a cool, dark place to prevent the essential oils from breaking down.

With a bit of trial and error and a dash of creativity, you'll soon be creating a fragrance to reflect every mood or that one special "signature scent" that others will remember you by.

When it comes to creating a pleasing fragrance, not all essential oils are created equal. Although beneficial for therapeutic purposes, some essential oils have a medicinal odor. Others can smell like turpentine. The essential oils listed in Table 8.2 are the most common scents used in perfumery. Once you understand the properties of each, you'll be able to shop for the perfect natural perfume or create one of your own.

Homemade Fragrance

Creating your own fragrance products is an exercise in self-expression. You can infuse your scent with essential oils to provide therapeutic benefits or blend components that reflect your personality to create a fragrance that is uniquely yours.

Table 8.2 ✿ Essential Oils for Perfumery

Essential Oil	Scent	Note	Aromatherapy Use	Comments and Cautions
bergamot	citrus	top	calming	may be a photosensitizer
bois de rose	sweet, floral	top	calming	
cedarwood	sweet, floral	middle	improves mental clarity	
chamomile	fruity	top	calming	
clary-sage	sweet, herbal	middle	calming	
clove	spicy	middle	uplifting	potential irritant
frankincense	fresh, balsamic	base	calming	
geranium	sweet, floral	middle	reduces anxiety	
grapefruit	citrus	top	energizing	
jasmine	floral, woodsy	base	none	usually extracted by solvents
lavender	fresh, herbal	top	reduces anxiety	
lemon	citrus	top	uplifting	
lemongrass	citrus	middle	stimulating	
lime	citrus	top	stimulating	
mandarin	citrus	top	calming	
myrrh	smoky, balsamic	base	calming	
neroli	citrus	middle	relieves tension	
palmarosa	sweet, floral	middle	calming	
patchouli	heavy, earthy	base	aphrodisiac	
peppermint	minty	top	energizing	
petitgrain	citrus	top	calming	

Essential Oil	Scent	Note	Aromatherapy Use	Comments and Cautions
rose	sweet, floral	middle	calming	
sandalwood	sweet, woody	base	calming	
spearmint	minty	top	energizing	
tangerine	citrus	middle	calming	
vanilla	sweet, smoky	base	calming	
vetiver	heavy, earthy	base	relieves tension	
ylang-ylang	heavy, floral	base	aphrodisiac	

Perfumes

Perfumes based on pure plant oils are more intense and last longer than colognes. Use them sparingly on your pulse points. These perfumes improve with age.

Citrus Morning
YIELD: 2 ounces

A refreshing fragrance with floral undertones. Perfect for a light, daytime scent.

> 5 drops grapefruit essential oil
> 4 drops lemongrass essential oil
> 3 drops jasmine essential oil
> 2 drops sandalwood essential oil
> 2 ounces grape seed oil

Blend the ingredients in a small dark-color glass bottle.

Evening Melody
YIELD: 1 ounce

A romantic perfume for those special evenings.

> 10 drops sandalwood essential oil
> 3 drops rose essential oil
> 1 ounce jojoba oil

Blend the ingredients in a small dark-color glass bottle.

Exotica
YIELD: 2 ounces

A deliciously mystical blend of essential oils from around the world.

> 12 drops frankincense essential oil
> 6 drops cedarwood essential oil
> 4 drops jasmine essential oil
> 2 drops neroli essential oil
> 2 ounces jojoba oil

Blend the ingredients in a small dark-color glass bottle.

Siren Song
YIELD: 1 ounce

A subtle, sexy fragrance. Patchouli and ylang-ylang blend with lavender to create a sensual fragrance designed to get attention.

> 6 drops cedarwood essential oil
> 4 drops lavender essential oil
> 2 drops ylang-ylang essential oil
> 1 drop patchouli essential oil
> 1 ounce jojoba oil

Blend the ingredients in a small dark-color glass bottle.

Spice
YIELD: 2 ounces

Wrap yourself in the mysteries of the Orient with this warm, spicy blend.

> 5 drops bergamot essential oil
> 5 drops mandarin essential oil
> 5 drops sandalwood essential oil
> 3 drops myrrh essential oil
> 3 drops clove essential oil
> 1 drop jasmine essential oil
> 2 ounces jojoba oil

Blend the ingredients in a small dark-color glass bottle.

Victorian Rose
YIELD: 2 ounces

Reminiscent of rose gardens and antique lace, this fragrance has a feminine floral scent.

3 drops bois de rose essential oil

2 drops rose essential oil

1 drop ylang-ylang essential oil

2 ounces grape seed oil

Blend the ingredients in a small dark-color glass bottle.

Colognes

The term *eau de cologne* is French for "water of Cologne." Although original formulas used alcohol to dilute the oils, the following scents use water for a light, airy cologne. These colognes improve as they age.

Lemon Lift

YIELD: 4 ounces

A crisp, clean scent with stimulating properties.

10 drops bergamot essential oil

5 drops lemongrass essential oil

3 drops grapefruit essential oil

3 drops tangerine essential oil

2 drops sandalwood essential oil

4 ounces distilled water

Combine the ingredients in an atomizer bottle and shake well to blend. Store in a cool, dark place, and shake daily for one week to allow the water to become infused with the oils.

Lavender Dreams

YIELD: 4 ounces

Lavender is traditionally used in aromatherapy to soothe stress.

10 drops lavender essential oil

4 drops bergamot essential oil

2 drops cedarwood essential oil

4 ounces distilled water

Combine the ingredients in an atomizer bottle and shake well to blend. Store in a cool, dark place, and shake daily for one week to allow the water to become infused with the oils.

Springtime Splash

YIELD: 4 ounces

Celebrate spring with this natural herbal cologne. Not as sweet as a floral blend, this cologne is light and refreshing.

15 drops lavender essential oil
10 drops chamomile essential oil
5 drops clary-sage essential oil
3 drops frankincense essential oil
4 ounces distilled water

Combine the ingredients in an atomizer bottle and shake well to blend. Store in a cool, dark place, and shake daily for one week to allow the water to become infused with the oils.

Winterwood

YIELD: 4 ounces

A warm, woodsy cologne slightly heavier than most floral blends. A perfect way to cure those winter blues.

15 drops cedarwood essential oil
10 drops bergamot essential oil
8 drops sandalwood essential oil
6 drops lavender essential oil
4 drops clary-sage essential oil
4 drops neroli essential oil
3 drops rose essential oil
4 ounces distilled water

Combine the ingredients in an atomizer bottle and shake well to blend. Store in a cool, dark place, and shake daily for one week to allow the water to become infused with the oils.

Scented Waters

Similar to colognes in their consistency, scented waters are a simple blend of water and a single essential oil. Often called floral waters, these products can also be used to scent your sheets and lingerie.

Basic Formula for Scented Water

YIELD: 4 ounces

Scented waters lend themselves to lighter floral and citrus oils rather than the heavier, earthy scents. Bois de rose, chamomile, lavender, lemon, and rose all make good choices. Since the aroma of each of these oils varies in strength, begin by adding 15 drops, adjusting upward to intensify the fragrance.

> 15 to 25 drops essential oil of your choice
> 4 ounces distilled water

Combine the ingredients in a spray bottle. Shake well to blend.

Enfleurage

This technique for extracting the essence of fresh flowers has been practiced by thrifty European women for generations. Although the traditional method uses an animal fat, such as lard, to absorb the fragrance, these two methods rely on vegetable compounds to achieve the same goal.

Floral Pomade   YIELD: 48 ounces

This is close to the traditional method and will produce a solid perfumed pomade. Although this is a wonderful way to preserve the scent of a flower garden, there are no exact measurements, and it is a time-consuming process.

> 6 cups vegetable shortening
> 6 cups fresh flower petals for each flower change

Melt enough pure vegetable shortening to cover the bottom of six large shallow glass plates to a depth of ½ inch (shallow pie plates work well). The plates must be the same size since they will be placed one on top of another in pairs. Pour the shortening into three of the plates. Allow the shortening to solidify, and then score it in a crisscross pattern with a sharp knife. Completely fill three of the plates with highly scented fresh flower petals, mounding the petals until the plates can hold no more. Place a plate over each of the flower-filled plates and seal together with masking tape to make an airtight container.

After a day or two, unseal the plates and remove the wilted petals. Repeat the process with fresh petals. When you have made seven or eight flower changes, cut up the shortening and pack it into several small containers with tight-fitting lids. To use, smooth a small amount onto your pulse points.

Perfume Oil   Yield: 4 ounces

This is a simple way to extract the fragrance of flowers that are too delicate to survive mechanical processing. Jasmine, lilac, and gardenia are ideal candidates for this type of extraction. Although the end result is not as concentrated as an essential oil, it is suitable for creating natural perfumes and colognes.

4 cups fresh flower petals
½ cup sunflower oil

Fill a clean 8-ounce glass jar with the flower petals, leaving 2 inches of head-space. Cover the petals completely with the oil (you may need to use additional oil). Cap with a tight-fitting lid and set the jar out in the sun. Allow it to sit for 24 hours.

Strain the oil into a small bowl and reserve. Discard the petals. Rinse the jar, making sure all plant material has been removed, and refill with 2 more cups of fresh petals. Pour the reserved oil over the petals, cap it, and set it out in the sun for another 24 hours. Repeat this process for several days, until you have a scent you are happy with. Store the finished fragrance oil in a cool, dark place. This oil can be used either undiluted or as part of a perfume mixture.

Sachets

Sachets are a wonderful way to scent lingerie, especially for those who enjoy fragrance but would rather not apply it directly to their skin.

Sachets can be made using small muslin spice bags, cheesecloth, a pretty bit of fabric tied with a ribbon, or tea bag papers available at health food stores. Use your imagination when combining herbs and flowers for a sachet. Here are a few formulas to get you started.

Jasmine Rose   Yield: 5½ cups

This blend uses a combination of fresh flowers and essential oils. As the flowers dry inside the sachet, they release their scent. Tuck these sachets into lingerie drawers, or drape them over the hangers of your favorite outfits.

4 cups rose petals
1 cup jasmine flowers

¼ cup orris root
¼ cup crushed cinnamon stick
10 drops each sandalwood, jasmine, and frankincense essential oil
4 drops patchouli essential oil

Combine the ingredients in a large bowl and mix well to disperse the essential oils. Pour 1 to 2 tablespoons of the mix into each sachet bag and secure tightly.

Sweet Vanilla   YIELD: 3 cups
This is a more sophisticated scent. The dried herbs can be purchased from an herb supplier.

2 cups dried sweet woodruff
½ cup vetiver root
2 vanilla beans, crushed
½ cup orris root
5 drops lime essential oil

Combine the ingredients in a large bowl and mix well to disperse the essential oil. Pour 1 to 2 tablespoons of the mix into each sachet bag and secure tightly.

Simple Lavender Sachet   YIELD: 3 cups
Quick and easy, this sachet will delicately scent your underthings. For a special bedtime treat, tuck a few sachets into your linen closet to scent your bedclothes.

2 cups dried lavender flowers
½ cup dried chamomile flowers
½ cup orris root
10 drops lavender essential oil

Combine the ingredients in a large bowl and mix well to disperse the essential oil. Pour 1 to 2 tablespoons of the mix into each sachet bag and secure tightly.

❧ Smart Shopping ☙

The right scent can calm frazzled nerves, inflame passion, or make you feel fresh and flirty. And when you choose a fragrance created without synthetics, you can indulge without worrying about how your scent impacts your health.

It shouldn't come as a surprise that the number of natural perfumes and colognes is limited. In a world where chemicals clutter department stores and drugstores, natural scents traditionally have been a tiny niche market available only at health food stores and through online or mail-order companies. But you can easily expand your fragrance options if you include scented waters and essential oils. Just remember to check the label to make sure the ingredients are pure and unadulterated.

Perfumes

Manufacturer	Product
Aubrey Organics	Angelica
	Elysian Fields
	Wild Wind

Colognes

Manufacturer	Product
Aubrey Organics	Lemon Blossom Body Splash
	Musk Splash

Scented Waters

Manufacturer	Product
Dreaming Earth Botanicals	Flower Waters
Green Valley Aromatherapy	Floral Waters
V'tae Parfum & Body Care	Parfum Waters

Perfume Balms and Pomades

Manufacturer	Product
Auric Blends	Temple Essence Perfume Solids
Birch Hill Happenings	Perfume Balms

Dynamo House	Meditation Balm
	Slow Down Balm
Terry and Co.	Yakshi Fragrances

Essential Oils

Manufacturer	Product
Adriaflor	Limited offering of organic essential oils; woman-owned company
Altered States Herbs	Pure essential oils
Aroma-Pure	Pure essential oils
Aura Cacia	Pure essential oils
Birch Hill Happenings	Pure essential oils
Camden-Grey	Pure essential oils
Dreaming Earth Botanicals	Organic and wild-crafted essential oils
Dynamo House	Limited selection of essential oils
Green Valley Aromatherapy	Pure essential oils
Indigo Wild	Pure essential oils
Jeanne Rose Aromatherapy	Pure essential oils
Mountain Rose Herbs	Pure essential oils
Natural Apothecary of Vermont	Certified organic essential oils
Rainbow Meadow	Pure essential oils
Spirit Scents	Pure essential oils
Tisserand	Pure essential oils

9

The Sacred Ritual: Cosmetics

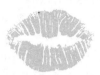

"The ceruse or white Lead wherewith women used to paint themselves was, without doubt, brought in use by the divell."
—Thomas Tuke, *A Treatise Against Painting and Tincturing of Men and Women*

Imagine a world of perpetual winter, where everything—trees, flowers, sea, and sky—is painted in shades of gray. Like the monochromatic mood of a 1950s B movie, a world without the counterpoint of color would be drab indeed. Color enriches our lives and sparks our creativity. Color can also enhance our looks.

For many of us, our first brush with color cosmetics came in early childhood, when we dabbled with our mothers' lipstick. It was our introduction to a rainbow of hues that would captivate us for the rest of our lives. As our intoxication became a habit, we began to rely on our daily dose of color to boost our confidence and even define who we were. Over the years, we've learned that a flick of a brush can minimize faults, enhance our bone structure, and even change our persona.

This fascination with color cosmetics isn't a new phenomenon. Archaeologists have traced color cosmetics back as far as the fourth millennium B.C. And, although early cosmetics were based on natural ingredients, they weren't necessarily safe. The ancient Egyptians used kohl, a poisonous compound made of antimony, to emphasize their eyebrows, eyelids, and lashes. And the Greeks and Romans painted their faces with white lead and chalk to achieve that classic pale complexion.

Cosmetics took a hiatus during the Dark Ages as Christianity gained popularity. According to the church, cosmetics were sinful, falling into the same league as idolatry and adultery. But, by the Renaissance, vanity won out over piety. Women once again returned to their "wicked ways"—often with deadly results. Pale skin was still the rage and could be achieved with a foundation of ceruse, a potent mixture of white lead and vinegar, applied to the face, neck, and bosom. Color was added to the cheeks and lips with vermilion, a highly toxic red face paint based on mercuric sulfide. Keeping the whole look in place required a heavy dose of powder, which was often based on talc.

Although the women weren't aware at the time that these toxic compounds were accumulating in their bodies, they did observe that the heavy coatings of lead caused a variety of skin problems. To regain the soft, fresh skin of youth, many women relied on lemon juice or rose water to treat the damage. Others, however, washed their faces with a popular facial peel made from mercury.

The pendulum swung back during the Victorian era, and the open use of cosmetics was once again frowned upon by respectable society; cosmetics were considered to be tools of the devil, more suited to prostitutes. The pristine look of innocence and virtue lasted until the end of the nineteenth century. But the dawn of the twentieth century brought sweeping changes. With the vote, women gained a degree of independence never before seen in America. One of the ways they expressed this newfound sense was with color cosmetics.

Although modern cosmetics weren't quite as deadly as those used in the past, women still didn't have an inkling of what their lipsticks and face powders contained. Neither did anyone else—except the manufacturers, who boldly told consumers that they didn't need to concern themselves with how the products were made. A 1935 Coty advertisement for lipstick even told women, "You don't, of course, care much about the making of a lipstick."[1] By 1940, scientists assured consumers that coal tar was one of the most remarkable and valuable substances on earth.[2] But with the passage of the Wheeler-Lea Act of 1938, better known as the Food, Drug, and Cosmetic Bill, the first small step in regulating the cosmetics industry had been taken.

The Color Controversy

In the early 1900s, cosmetics colors based on natural ingredients became replaced by chemically synthesized colors derived from aniline, a petroleum product that is toxic in its pure form. Known as "coal tar colors" because the starting material was obtained from bituminous coal, these synthetic colors were easy to produce, less expensive, and capable of providing consistent color that blended well with other ingredients. But as the use of synthetic colors grew, so did concern over their safety.

Before 1938, color additives fell under the jurisdiction of the Food and Drug Act of 1906. However, since the skin was assumed to be an impervious barrier, cosmetics were not included in this early attempt to ensure the safety of color additives. The act was refined in 1938 to include cosmetics, and the Food and Drug Administration (FDA) set about creating a premarket approval process for color additives. These new requirements were the beginning of a battle still being waged today over the color certification process.

Based on the new law, the FDA recommended the certification of seventeen coal tar colors in 1939 and created a numbering system for certified colors along with three classifications that are still in use today:

FD&C Colors: Colors certified for use in foods, drugs, and cosmetics.

D&C Colors: Additives considered safe for use in drugs and cosmetics that can be ingested or that come in direct contact with the mucous membranes.

Ext. D&C Colors: Dyes and pigments that are not considered safe for foods because of their oral toxicity but that have been deemed safe for use in drugs and cosmetics applied to the skin.

An amendment to the act, known as the Delaney Amendment, was passed in 1960 and banned any color additive found to cause cancer in humans or animals. The new law required food and chemical manufacturers to test colors for safety and stated that "no additive may be permitted in any amount if the tests show that it produces cancer when fed to man or animals or by other appropriate tests." Although the Delaney Amendment seemed all-inclusive at the time, the new requirement did not extend to cosmetics. After the amendment was passed, all colors currently in use, including those used in cosmetics, were placed on a provisional list until further testing could be done. Even though the provisional list was supposed to be temporary, many of the colors used today still remain on the list—colors whose safety has not been proved or even studied.

Certified colors must undergo batch testing by the FDA to make sure they fall within the specifications set for each color. Limitations are placed on each certifiable color additive for the level of impurities it may legally contain. An entire batch may be rejected if the levels are discovered to be too high. Colors are also tested for acute oral toxicity, irritation, sensitizing potential, and subacute skin toxicity. However, the FDA commissioner can waive any of these tests based on the data submitted by the manufacturer.

In 1992, the agency rejected 40 of the 3,942 batches tested.[3] Other years contain periods when every batch analyzed was certified. For instance, during the first quarter of 2001, 3,364,734.63 pounds of color additives were analyzed, and the same amount was certified.[4] Not a single batch was found to be unacceptable. While proponents of the current system believe that such an incredible certification rate speaks to the safety of the synthetic colors contained in cosmetics, critics may wonder if these numbers are actually a reflection of an economic incentive to certify color additives since manufacturers must pay the FDA for every pound of color the agency certifies. The going rate is $154 for each pound tested but not less than $100 per batch. When a manufacturer petitions the FDA to test a new color additive, the company must also submit a deposit of $2,600. If a manufacturer wants to use a certified color for a purpose other than that specified by the FDA, it will cost the manufacturer $1,800 to amend the listing.[5]

Color additives used in cosmetics come in two forms: straight colors and lakes. Straight colors are certifiable colors that dissolve in water. Lakes are insoluble and are produced through the absorption of a water-soluble dye by a hydrated aluminum substrate. Lakes, although provisionally listed on the FDA's list of approved colors, are commonly used to tint eye shadow and lipsticks, products in which "bleeding" may be a problem. All lakes are subject to certification before being permanently listed.[6]

What about exempt colors? Since exempt colors originally derived from mineral or botanical sources, they are often considered natural, even though today's exempt colors are often chemically synthesized. In fact, iron oxide pigments are required to be synthesized before they can be used in cosmetics. While cosmetics manufacturers like to claim that exempt colors are "natural," those prepared synthetically are not naturally occurring.

Exempt colors must also meet certain specifications, much like their nonexempt counterparts, but aren't required to undergo batch testing to be certified. This means that, even though they are certified, some batches of exempt colors may be contaminated. Even if they aren't, the safety of some exempt colors is questionable. Twenty-nine exempt color additives are currently in use. Table 9.1 shows a few of the more popular "natural" colors in the typical makeup bag.

Table 9.1 🍃 "Natural" Colors

Exempt Color	Use	Comments and Cautions
aluminum powder	approved for externally applied cosmetics, including those used in the eye area; often contained in face powders	created from finely divided particles of aluminum; aluminum potentially linked to the development of Alzheimer's disease
bismuth oxychloride	approved for general cosmetic use; often contained in eye shadow	often called synthetic pearl; may cause allergic reactions
dihydroxyacetone	approved for externally applied cosmetics intended solely or in part to give color to the human body	obtained by the action of bacteria on glycerol; lethal to rats when injected in large doses; can cause contact dermatitis
manganese violet	approved for general cosmetic use; often contained in eye shadow	toxic when inhaled
mica	approved for general cosmetic use; adds a pearly luster and "slip" to face powders	derived from the muscovite mica; a respiratory irritant when inhaled

Despite the FDA's confidence in its testing methods, some synthetic colors that have been approved can promote acne or cause allergic contact dermatitis. And studies have shown all coal tar colors to cause cancer in animals. Although the FDA maintains that any cancer risk is minimal—as low as one in a billion, the World Health Organization has pointed out inconsistencies in the FDA's safety data.[7] For example, in 1990, all uses of the lakes of Red No. 3 were banned. However, the straight color, while banned for use in cosmetics because it was determined to be carcinogenic, is still permanently listed for use in foods and ingested drugs.[8]

Synthetic colors aren't the only ingredients that merit women's concern. Dubious chemicals can be identified in all types of color cosmetics. This chapter gives you the scoop, from the foundation up.

Shaky Foundations

For those of us with less-than-perfect complexions, a good foundation can be our best friend, giving us a healthy glow while covering up flaws and blemishes. Unfortunately, while foundations may cover up our skin's shortcomings, they are the third leading cause of contact dermatitis.[9]

The most popular base makeups are cream foundations. Pigmented to mimic our natural skin tones, these products are available in water-based, oil-based, oil-free, and long-lasting formulas. While a good base can help moisturize your skin and protect it from environmental pollutants, a foundation packed with synthetic chemicals can spell trouble, especially since these products remain on your skin all day. Along with the synthetic colors that give a product its particular tint, most conventional cream foundations contain mineral oil, which can block the pores and promote cosmetic acne. Lanolin, a known allergen, is another common ingredient. Although natural brands often use glycerin to carry moisture, most mainstream foundations rely on propylene glycol, a neurotoxin and skin sensitizer. Formaldehyde-releasing 2-bromo-2-nitropropane-1,3-diol and triethanolamine (TEA) are other chemicals frequently found together in base makeups—a dangerous combination that may cause the formation of nitrosamines.

Stick foundations are a relatively new addition to the cosmetics counter and a convenient way to touch up your foundation or cover blemishes. But this convenience has a downside. Along with their mineral oil, beeswax, and synthetic fragrance, stick foundations contain isopropyl myristate, a fatty compound that can cause blackheads. More worrisome is the fact that, if the product is contaminated with NDELA (n-nitrosodiethanolamine), carcinogenic nitrosamines may be formed and readily absorbed into the skin when isopropyl myristate is present.

Of all the preservatives manufacturers include in liquid and stick foundations, the parabens seem to be particular favorites. Potentially hormone-disrupting preservatives that may accumulate in body fat, parabens are also frequent allergens. Another preservative often included in foundations is quaternium-15, a germicide that may break down into formaldehyde.

For a healthier foundation, look for natural brands that rely on iron oxides and titanium dioxide instead of FD&C and D&C colors. These products also replace the mineral oil with natural plant oils for cover without the chemicals.

Concealing the Truth

While foundations are designed to give you a flawless canvas upon which to apply the rest of your makeup, there are times when foundation just isn't enough. Dark circles, blemishes, and age spots can require the heavy-duty cover provided by concealers. Available in creams, sticks, or brush-on formulations, concealers can be fairly thin or quite thick, but one thing conventional concealers all have in common is the number of irritating chemicals in them. Commonly used ingredients such as propylene glycol and lanolin may be sensitizers and allergens, as can paraben preservatives. Other preservatives often used in concealers include imidazolidinyl urea, the second most reported cause of contact dermatitis, and BHA, a carcinogen that can be absorbed through the skin.

If you use a foundation with good coverage, you may be able to forgo a concealer altogether. If you must use these products, check the ingredients listed on the label before purchasing. Natural brands rely on plant oils and waxes, kaolin, and iron oxides instead of irritants and carcinogens to disguise flaws.

Powder Puffery

Once the foundation and concealer are applied, most women opt for a dusting of powder to hold everything in place and give them a finished look. How safe are these facial powders? One concern is that, as the powder sets up, it can block the pores and prevent the skin's natural respiration. Another is that, once the product is airborne—a particular problem with loose powders—it constitutes a respiratory threat due to the high volume of talc. Some powders also include formaldehyde releasers such as 2-bromo-2-nitropropane-1,3-diol and quaternium-15, along with myriad paraben preservatives.

For a nontoxic alternative, look for a powder based on cornstarch, kaolin, or silk powder and colored with titanium dioxide, iron oxides, or botanicals such as cinnamon and henna. If you have fair skin and suffer from color-related allergies or don't need the additional color provided by commercial powders, a light dusting of plain old cornstarch will give your makeup a translucent finish.

A Brush with Blush

It's a sad fact that as we age, we lose the healthy glow of youth. Blush to the rescue! Depending on the shade, blush can put the "roses" back in our cheeks or shade areas we would like to diminish. The skillful application of blush can also create a sophisticated look by giving us those haughty cheekbones for which fashion models are famous. Here, too, while blush gives us the illusion of health, there's nothing healthy about the ingredients in mainstream brands.

Talc is the primary ingredient in most conventional blushes—comprising up to 50 percent of some brands. Although some of the safer iron oxides and ultramarines could achieve the same effect, synthetic colors are used to lend that luscious hue to the product, particularly D&C Red No. 33 and FD&C Yellow Nos. 5 and 6. To get all that color neatly pressed into an attractive compact requires at least one binder, such as mineral oil or propylene glycol, and thickeners. The most common thickening agents are the acrylate compounds, chemicals that can be strong irritants.[10]

Fortunately, you can create a healthy glow without exposing yourself to these potentially dangerous toxins. Opt instead for color based on natural coloring agents and bentonite or kaolin clay for a blush that is as healthy as the illusion it creates.

Jeepers Peepers!

The eyes are our most expressive feature. It's only natural to want to play them up with a colorful palate of cosmetics! But chemical-filled eye shadows, liners, and mascaras can turn our most intriguing asset into a painful eyesore and may lead to some long-term health problems.

Eye shadow offers consumers a fantasyland of colors, from electric blue to metallic gold to smoky charcoal, and typically comes in two forms: powder or cream. Although the FDA has banned the use of some coal tar colors in eye makeup,[11] conventional eye shadows still contain a cast of shady characters. Common coal tar derivatives present in mainstream eye shadow include the lakes of FD&C Blue No. 1, a frequent allergen, and FD&C Yellow No. 5, which may cause severe reactions in people allergic to aspirin. It's estimated that between 47,000 and 94,000 nonallergic consumers are also sensitive to this particular dye.[12] FD&C Red No. 40 Aluminum Lake, one of the newest colors available to manufacturers, is also a frequent addition to eye shadow. This color was approved for use around the eye area in 1994, despite controversy over the fact that all the safety testing was done by the manufacturer. Based on animal studies, the National Cancer Institute has reported that p-credine, a chemical used in the manufacturing of FD&C Red No. 40, is carcinogenic.[13]

As with blush, powdered eye shadow's main component is talc. Mineral oil and dimethicone, a silicone oil, are also added to help the powder adhere to the eyelid. Binding the talc and oils are ingredients such as polymethyl methacrylate, a binder and film-forming component that is a strong irritant.

Are cream eye shadows any healthier? Hardly! Cream eye shadows are typically packed with petrochemicals such as petrolatum and paraffin, along with the same FD&C colors prevalent in their powdered cousins. Lanolin, a frequent allergen, is also included. Along with the traditional hues, cream eye shadows also come in glittery, iridescent colors that are created by adding pure aluminum. While they can be fun to wear, eye shadows that contain particles of glitter are capable of producing violent allergic reactions. Moreover, stray particles may enter the eye and result in injuries to the cornea.

One tiny container of eye shadow can hold three or more preservatives, including quaternium-15 and imidazolidinyl urea. Methyl- and propyl-parabens are also frequently used, despite research that has linked parabens to severe allergic reactions in up to 1 percent of the population.[14]

A study from Helsinki, Finland, brings more frightening news. Researchers at the Consumer Agency and Ombudsman tested forty-nine eye shadows for the presence of lead, cobalt, nickel, chromium, and arsenic. All the samples were determined to contain at least one part per million and up to forty-nine parts per million of at least one of these elements.[15] Although the researchers didn't feel that these levels would cause anything more serious than occasional allergic reactions and sensitivities, new research from Dartmouth College shows that chronic exposure to very low levels of arsenic—lower than those found in the Finnish study—are capable of hormonal disruption.[16]

Avoiding these irritants and allergens may seem impossible, but natural manufacturers have devised a way to color your lids without synthetics. They rely on cornstarch, kaolin, titanium dioxide, and iron oxides. In addition, although many natural eye shadows do contain parabens, some brands prevent spoilage instead with a dose of vitamin E—an effective alternative to synthetic preservatives.

Now that your eyelids are delicately tinted, do you automatically reach for the eyeliner? Today you can choose from an eyeliner pencil for a softly smudged look or a liquid liner for sharper definition. Whichever type you choose, lining your eyes may expose them to alkanolamines such as TEA, synthetic pigments, and polyvinylpyrrolidone (PVP). Long used in hair sprays, PVP was recently identified as a cosmetics allergen by researchers in France.[17] What's more, there is limited evidence that PVP causes cancer in laboratory animals.[18]

According to the American Medical Association, many consumers have suffered swelling and irritation after using eyeliners. Further, numerous instances of bacterial contamination in liquid eyeliners have been documented by the FDA. The agency has also received a significant number of reports citing allergic reactions to these products.[19] A gentler and safer alternative is to choose one of the many natural eye pencils made of plant waxes and iron oxides.

Mascara is another problematic product. While we all love long, lush lashes, a glance at the ingredients listed on most conventional mascaras can really curl your eyelashes! Petroleum distillates, shellac, and acrylates are common ingredients of major brands. Phenylmercuric acetate, a preservative derived from benzene and mercury, is another frequent addition and may cause allergic reactions, skin irritation, and blisters. Heavy on paraben preservatives, mainstream mascaras may also contain quaternium-22, a preservative that can cause contact allergies.[20] More serious is the addition of pentaerythrityl, a resin additive made from acetaldehyde and formaldehyde.

What about those "lash-extending" formulas? Many brands contain plasticizers such as polyisobutene and polyurethane or the plasticlike compounds of aluminum stearates to achieve those great lengths. Not only do these chemicals harden your lashes, making them prone to breakage, but also, some plasticizers, such as polyurethane, have been found to cause cancer in animals.[21] Lash-building mascaras can also contain sodium polystyrene sulfonate, a chemical used to manufacture cosmetics resins. While polystyrene can irritate the eyes, some researchers see an even darker side to this plasticizer after identifying it as a nonylphenol that behaves like estrogen.[22]

Fortunately, nontoxic mascaras are available in black, brown, and even navy. Made with plant waxes and oils, herbs, vitamins, and iron oxides, these natural lash builders are just as effective as their chemical counterparts. But even natural mascara can cause problems if you're not careful. Because of their design, mascara wands can scratch the eye, leading to bacterial infections such as conjunctivitis.

Lethal Lips

Lipstick is the finishing touch that makes your face come alive. Whether we choose a delicate pink, a warm rust, or a lusty red, lipstick provides a polished look that pulls the rest of your makeup together. The right lipstick can also moisturize and condition the lips to keep them soft and sensuous—a challenge since our lips have no oil glands and are more sensitive to the elements than other parts of the body.

Can drugstore and department store lipsticks offer the kind of protection our lips need to keep them kissable? Mainstream lipsticks are a blend of synthetic oils, such as mineral oil, and petroleum waxes, along with pigments. One of the most frequent ingredients, a plasticlike wax known as microcrystalline wax, may cause allergic reactions. Other allergens commonly contained in lipstick are amyldimethylamino benzoic acid, ricinoleic acid, fragrance, ester gums, and lanolin.

Then there are the colors. Lipsticks sport more synthetic pigments than any other type of cosmetic—representing a veritable who's who of coal tar colors. While many authorities believe that all coal tar derivatives are carcinogenic, some of these colors can result in immediate problems. FD&C Yellow Nos. 5 and 6 have been surrounded by controversy for years because of their potential to cause allergic reactions. And eosin dyes, such as D&C Orange No. 5 and D&C Red No. 27, may cause photosensitivity and cheilitis, a form of dermatitis that makes the lips cracked, dry, and inflamed. It's been said that, over the course of a lifetime, a woman will ingest more than four pounds of lipstick! If you wear lipstick every day, the total may be higher. Each time we lick our lips, eat, drink, or chew on our lips while wearing lipstick, we consume more of these dubious chemicals.

If conventional lipsticks have you seeing red, don't think that switching to a mainstream lip gloss will protect you from toxins. Although the manufacturers of lip gloss and lip balms would like you to believe that their products will moisturize and protect your lips, it's doubtful that synthetic waxes and oils can actually penetrate the skin on the lips. What may be absorbed by your lips is phenol, a common ingredient in lip balms. Phenol is a poisonous substance that can be absorbed through the skin. Exposure by skin absorption or ingestion of even a small amount can cause nausea, vomiting, convulsions, paralysis, collapse of the circulatory system, and even death. Minute amounts can result in skin rashes, swelling, pimples, and hives.[23]

The latest trend in lip gloss is the addition of sunscreen. Benzophenones are frequently added to protect your lips from ultraviolet light. These chemicals, which have been linked to hives and contact sensitivity,[24] may act as a weak xeno-estrogen, according to a recent study by the Tokyo Metropolitan Research Laboratory of Public Health.[25]

If the chemicals in these seemingly benign products make you shudder, the ingredients in lip gloss designed for children can read like a toxic horror story. One popular product among the seven- to ten-year-old set is Bonne Bell's Jewel Lips Lip Smacker. Tucked into the colorful tube promising glitter gloss and a fruity taste are a slew of ingredients to which no child should be exposed. Phthalic anhydride, a moderate irritant made from naphthalene, is a prominent ingredient in the product. Short-term dermal exposure to napthalene can result in headaches, nausea, vomiting, diarrhea, confusion, convulsions, and coma and has been linked to kidney damage and brain damage in infants. Although the Environmental Protection Agency does not classify napthalene as a human carcinogen, there is some evidence from animal studies that it causes fetal and maternal toxicity.[26] Allergy-inducing plasticizers such as microcrystalline wax and polyisobutene are also listed on the ingredient label. Rounding out the product are petrolatum, polyacryladipate, propylparabens, synthetic flavor, and a variety of FD&C and D&C colors. On the Bonne Bell website, the company proudly announces that it does not test on animals. It's a shame it doesn't share the same concern for our children.

Do we really need all these petroleum derivatives to attain luscious lips? No, say natural cosmetics manufacturers. Instead, look for lip colors and conditioners that are based on beeswax, plant oils, vitamin E, and iron oxides.

One note on natural lipsticks: Since they do not rely on chemical waxes, they are softer than drugstore and department store brands. They also have a tendency to melt at lower temperatures, so don't leave them lying around in your glove compartment or in direct sunlight.

A Permanent Solution?

Some women prefer to avoid the cosmetics counter all together, opting instead for "permanent" makeup. The pitch sounds tempting: you can look good 24/7, even when you wake up in the morning. And think of all the time and money you could save without the daily routine of "putting on your face." Alas, no matter how terrific permanent makeup sounds, it's a practice that can leave you vulnerable to some serious health risks.

Permanent cosmetic makeup is actually a form of tattooing, depositing color additives directly into the dermis, the middle layer of the skin. It's an invasive procedure that requires the use of needles to apply the color. None of the inks used, however, have been approved by the FDA for injection into the skin. According to the FDA, using an unapproved color additive in a tattoo ink adulterates the ink. In fact, many of the pigments used in tattoo inks are not approved for skin contact at all but only for industrial use such as printers' ink and automobile paint.[27] And, as in any form of permanent tattooing, these pigments fade over time and require periodic touch-ups.

Although some salons claim to be certified in the art of permanent makeup, according to San Francisco's Pacific Tattoo, there is no true certification available to practitioners. Too often, practitioners in salons offering permanent makeup have acquired their training at a school that lasts only a few days or through a home training course or video. A major problem with using an unskilled practitioner is that he or she may place the dye too deeply into the skin, a mistake that can cause the dye to "bleed" into the surrounding tissue.[28] Even if you find a practitioner with a high level of skill and years of experience, complications can occur. Common problems include infection, allergic reactions, and scarring. The most serious consequence of permanent makeup can result from using needles that have not been properly sterilized. Since a bacterial disease or blood-borne virus, including hepatitis or HIV,[29] can be transferred from an infected person to the client, the use of unsterilized equipment can put a client's life at risk.

Tinting or dying the eyelashes, another service offered by some salons, is a procedure that has caused a great deal of concern at the FDA. Permanent hair dye is often used to get the job done, even though these products have not been approved for use around the eyes. Although the agency has no authority to regulate the practice, it warns consumers that this practice can result in eye injury and even blindness.[30]

If you decide, despite the risks, that you still want permanent makeup, ask yourself this: what if you don't like the way the makeup looks once it's been applied, or you tire of it a few years later? Permanent makeup can be removed, but the procedure is costly and time-consuming. The most successful method of removal is with lasers. However, treating permanently lined eyes and lips can occasionally cause a reaction that turns the original color to black.[31] Even if things go smoothly, the permanent makeup that cost $400 to $800 to apply will cost upward of $3,000 to remove.

Some women, regardless of the risk, will continue to apply toxins to their faces or undergo dangerous procedures in the name of beauty. But if you've made it this far, you're probably not among them. It's time to reward yourself and enjoy the healthy and beautiful natural products you've chosen to enhance your own beauty ritual.

Makeup Magic

Makeup is supposed to be fun. Now that you've thrown away all those drugstore and department store lipsticks and eye shadows—and replaced them with wholesome, nontoxic cosmetics from your local health food store—it's time to play!

When it comes to makeup, most women fall into one of two categories. The first are women who are basically comfortable with the look they've developed over the years. They know what colors they like and rarely veer from the norm. The other group consists of makeup junkies who follow each new trend as if it were manna from heaven. Each season's new colors bring the opportunity to try something new, to re-create their "look." But the art of makeup has less to do with the colors you use than with how the products are applied. If you are still using the techniques you learned when you were in high school, it's time for a refresher course in basic makeup application.

Like anything else in life, when it comes to applying makeup, there are some rules that shouldn't be broken:

- Always start with a scrupulously clean face. As any artist knows, a clean canvas is essential for a beautiful outcome.
- Prime your face with a good, natural moisturizer.
- Always use the best tools you can afford. Good-quality natural-bristle makeup brushes give you not only more control but also a more natural, longer-lasting result.
- Keep your tools clean. A weekly soak in soapy water will prevent the accumulation of bacteria, dust, and dead skin cells.
- Unless you aspire to looking like Tammy Faye Bakker, remember that your makeup should always look natural. Your face is the first thing people notice. Even if it takes you an hour to apply your makeup, you want people to see you, not your paint job.
- As we get older, our hair lightens, and our skin tone changes. The colors you sported in your teens and twenties can look harsh and unnatural in your forties and fifties. Opt for more-neutral colors that match or coordinate with your skin tone.
- Use a light touch, particularly as you age. A heavy hand accentuates fine lines and wrinkles.

Regardless of what you've heard at the cosmetics counter, when it comes to color cosmetics, you need only a handful of products to achieve a classic, well-groomed look: foundation, concealer, powder, blush, eye shadow, mascara, and lipstick. You may want to add eyeliner or a lip pencil to your repertoire, but it's not absolutely necessary.

Now that you know the rules and have the tools, it's time to begin.

Foundation

Buying the right foundation is the first step toward creating a beautifully natural look. To avoid ending up with an obvious makeup job, you'll want to match the foundation to your natural skin color. How can you tell if that tawny bottle of foundation is the right one for you? Instead of testing the product on the back of your hand, smooth a bit on your neck or jawline. Unless the store offers an abundance of natural light, walk out into the sun and check your mirror. If you can see an obvious color difference, it's the wrong shade for you.

Water-based foundations provide sheer, natural coverage without emphasizing fine lines. For a light, seamless look, apply the foundation all over your face with a clean, damp cosmetic sponge. Don't forget your eyelids! Then blend, blend, blend the product over your skin, up to your hairline, and just under your jawline. Blending your foundation not only gives you the lightest coverage possible but also helps prevent streaking.

Concealer

Next comes the concealer. No matter what your age, a good concealer can cover up blemishes, age spots, and those dark circles under your eyes. Whether you prefer a stick or cream, choose a shade slightly lighter than your natural skin tone. Dab a bit of the concealer on the area you wish to camouflage, and blend it thoroughly into your foundation with your makeup sponge to prevent a "two-tone" look.

Powder

Now that your face is flawless, you'll want to keep it that way with a natural facial powder. A loose, translucent powder, in a shade that closely matches your foundation, will give your makeup staying power. Using a dry, fluffy brush designed for powder, lightly dust the powder over your entire face, making sure you remove any excess.

Blush

Your canvas is now ready for blush. The right blush can give you a youthful, healthy glow. Be sure to keep the color natural. Forget blushes with brown or red overtones. Opt instead for a warm pink or peach.

Drag your brush lightly over the blush, and then blow off the excess to prevent a stripe of concentrated color from being deposited on your cheeks. Now smile and apply the blush lightly over the apple of your cheek (you can always apply more if necessary). Sweep the blush toward the hairline, feathering the edges to blend.

Eye Shadow

Now comes the step many women consider to be the most fun, yet it is also the part that causes the most anxiety—the eyes. Since the eyes are the focal point of the face, it's only natural that we want to avoid mistakes. A steady hand and some practice are all it takes to achieve professional results, particularly when it comes to eye shadow.

If you want professional results, the type of eye shadow you choose can make all the difference. Cream shadows have a tendency to smear and collect in the creases of your eyelid. For lasting color that stays where you put it, look for natural pressed-powder eye shadows. Choose three fairly neutral colors—light, medium, and dark. Avoid the neon blues and greens that were popular in the 1970s, and don't make the mistake of thinking that your shadow needs to match your eye color or your outfit. Opt instead for shades of brown and beige. If these seem a bit too conservative for your taste, a muted plum or olive can lend some color to your eyes while still appearing natural. One caution: Never use a sponge-tip applicator when applying eye shadow. They are a magnet for bacteria and offer far less control. Use natural-bristle brushes specifically designed for eye shadow. It may take a little practice, but once you get the hang of it, you'll wonder how you ever got by without them.

Applying eye shadow is a three-step procedure. First, using an eye shadow brush, apply the lightest color over the entire lid, from brow to lashes. Next, apply the medium tone to your lower lid, from the lashes to the crease. Finally, apply the darkest color to the crease, blending it slightly to avoid a defined line.

Setting Your Makeup

Once the foundation and all powdered cosmetics have been applied, many exclusive salons will spritz the client's face with a fine mist of imported (and expensive) water. Although you may think this practice simply helps to justify the high price tag of a makeover, there is a reason for this step. As the water drys, it helps "set" the makeup, helping it last longer. You can achieve the same effect without the expense by lightly misting your face with distilled water or one of the herbal mist formulas in Chapter 4.

Eyeliner

Once you've finished applying the dry cosmetics, it's time for eyeliner. Defining your eyes with eyeliner can frame your lashes and make them appear thicker. The trick is to apply the eyeliner so that it is barely noticeable. Thick black lines, "Cleopatra wings," and eyeliner under the lower lashes will give you a heavy, dated look. And, forget about lining the inside rim of the eyes, a trend that was popular in the 1980s. It's a surefire invitation to infection and injury. Instead, draw a fine line at the base of the eyelashes with a soft eyeliner pencil in charcoal gray or dark brown. Begin at the outer corner of your eyelid and draw the thinnest line possible, tapering it as you approach the inner corner. For the most natural look, gently smudge the line with a cotton swab.

Eyebrows

Eyebrows frame your eyes and give your face character. Keeping them well groomed is essential to creating a polished look. Although most of us can get away with a little policing and artful shaping, some women must contend with either too little or too much eyebrow hair. In such cases, a little cosmetic wizardry can bring balance to those brows.

Fill in sparse eyebrows with a soft eye pencil or a bit of eye shadow, choosing a color that closely matches your natural brow color. Apply with a light hand, using short, feathering strokes to avoid looking as if you've drawn on your brows with a crayon.

If your brows are unruly, tame them with a bit of aloe vera gel. Simply coat an eyebrow brush with the gel and lightly brush the hairs into place. As the gel dries, it keeps the hairs from straying, leaving you with neat, natural-looking eyebrows.

Mascara

Finish your eyes with a coat of mascara. Unless you are very blond, choose a soft black. For a more natural look, women with light blond hair should opt for a dark brown. Sweep the mascara from the root of the lashes to the tips, first on the underside and then on the tops. One coat should be enough to enhance your lashes. For the occasional clump, use an eyelash comb to separate the lashes and remove any excess mascara.

One problem many of us experience with mascara is that the tube never seems to last as long as it should. Within a month or two, the product becomes dried out and unusable. According to professional makeup artists, it's not the mascara's fault—it's ours. Their advice? Never pump the mascara wand. Doing so forces air into the tube and makes the mascara dry out prematurely. Instead, gently rotate the wand several times before removing it from the tube. Another tip: Never add water to the container to thin the mascara. Adding liquid will encourage bacterial growth. If your mascara becomes too thick, place the tube in warm water for several minutes to thin the consistency.

Lips

Making up your lips will give you a finished look, particularly if you choose a shade that complements your coloring. Since very few people can actually pull off blood red lips, experiment with soft reds, rusts, or pinks.

To give your lipstick a soft, smooth base, apply a lip fixative, such as a vitamin E stick. The vitamin E will also nourish your lips and help prevent chapping. If your lipstick has a habit of bleeding, outline your mouth with a lip pencil in a shade that closely matches your lipstick.

Finally, apply your lipstick. The best way is with a lip brush. Rub the brush on the lipstick, making sure to pick up a sufficient amount of color to fill in your lips. Start with the outer edges of the lips and work your way toward the inner edges with a back-and-forth motion. Most makeup artists recommend holding your mouth taut and slightly open to get the best coverage.

One practice that is a holdover from the 1950s is "blotting" your lips with a tissue after they have been made up. Under no circumstances should you blot your lipstick once it's been applied. The color will not last as long, and you will undermine the moist look of the lipstick.

Once you get the hang of professional makeup application, you should be able to apply your makeup in ten minutes or less. It's time well spent. By enhancing your natural beauty, you will give the world a glimpse of the beautiful spirit that lies within.

Unlike many of the other products in this book, most color cosmetics aren't based on herbs and can't be created at home. Instead, they rely on other nontoxic ingredients to gently lend color, texture, and substance to their products. Table 9.2 lists some of the best natural ingredients to look for when you go shopping.

Table 9.2 & Natural Cosmetics Ingredients

Ingredient	Characteristics	Found In
annatto	a natural yellow-to-pink vegetable dye	lipstick
beeswax	a by-product of bees; used as an emulsifier	stick concealer, lipstick, lip gloss, mascara
candelilla wax	obtained from candelilla plants	lipstick, mascara
carmine	a crimson pigment derived from the dried bodies of the cochineal insect	lipstick, blush
carrageenan	a seaweed extract derived from Irish moss; used as a stabilizer and emulsifier	liquid foundation
cornstarch	a finely powdered corn flour obtained by wet milling	powder, blush, eye shadow
hematite	an earthy red, naturally occurring mineral	powder, blush
iron oxides	oxidized iron that varies in color; FDA requires all iron oxides be synthesized	liquid foundation, powder, blush, eye shadow, mascara, eyeliner, lipstick
jojoba oil	extracted from the seeds of the Simondsia chinensis plant; used as a lubricant	concealer, lipstick
kaolin	absorbent powder mined from Kaoling Hill in the Jiangxi Province in China	cake foundation, concealer, powder, blush

Ingredient	Characteristics	Found In
pycnogenol	antioxidant derived from the French maritime pine tree; used as a natural preservative	powder, blush, eye shadow, lipstick
rice bran oil	oil expressed from the rice grain	liquid foundation
shea butter	a natural fat obtained from the karite tree	lipstick
silk powder	coloring ingredient obtained from the secretion of silkworms	powder, blush
sunflower oil	obtained from sunflower seeds; an emollient rich in vitamin E	foundation, concealer
sweet almond oil	an emollient obtained from the *Prunus Amygdalus dulcis* tree	liquid foundation, concealer, lipstick
titanium dioxide	a naturally occurring mineral; used as a tinting powder	liquid foundation, powder, eyeliner, eye shadow, lipstick
vitamins A, C, and E	potent antioxidants that also serve as natural preservatives	most natural color cosmetics

❧ Smart Shopping ❦

Color cosmetics can give your self-image a boost and add pizzazz to your looks. But drugstore and department store brands can expose you to a plethora of synthetic colors and preservatives that can undermine your health.

Unfortunately, it is virtually impossible to create your own pure and natural color cosmetics at home. But you can buy them. Natural cosmetics companies offer color cosmetics in health food stores, through mail order, and via the Internet. But beware: Even if most of the ingredients are natural, some manufacturers still rely on synthetic preservatives. Read the labels carefully!

There are a few companies that make truly natural, preservative-free color cosmetics in a wide range of colors. To help simplify your search for nontoxic color cosmetics, look for the products listed here that are followed by an asterisk (*).

Foundation

Manufacturer	Product
Burt's Bees	Wings of Love Tinted Facial Moisturizer*
Dr. Hauschka	Colored Day Creams*
Gabriel	Dual Powder Foundation
	Moisturizing Liquid Foundation
Kiss My Face	Moisturizing Sheer Foundation
NaturElle	Dual Powder Foundation
	Matte Foundation
Perfectly Beautiful	Beauty Essentials Corrective Protective*
Real Purity	Creme Foundation*

Concealer

Manufacturer	Product
Burt's Bees	Wings of Love Concealing Creme*
Gabriel	Concealer
Paul Penders	Nutritious Color Cover-Up Stick*
Perfectly Beautiful	Beauty Essentials Concealer*
Real Purity	Concealer*

Powder

Manufacturer	Product
Aubrey Organics	Natural Translucent Base*
Burt's Bees	Wings of Love Facial Powder*
NaturElle	Mattiste Finishing Powder
	Sheer Tones

Blush

Manufacturer	Product
Aubrey Organics	Silken Earth*
Burt's Bees	Wings of Love Blushing Creme*
Dr. Hauschka	Cheek Colors*
Gabriel	Blush
NaturElle	Vibrance Blushers
Perfectly Beautiful	Beauty Essentials Blusher*
Real Purity	Powder Blush*

Eye Shadow

Manufacturer	Product
Dr. Hauschka	Eye Shadows*
Ecco Bella	Eye Shadow
Gabriel	Eye Shadow
NaturElle	Accent Eye Colours
Perfectly Beautiful	Beauty Essentials Eye Shadow

Eye Pencils

Manufacturer	Product
NaturElle	Ellegance Kohl Eyeliner

Mascara

Manufacturer	Product
Dr. Hauschka	Mascara*
Gabriel	Mascara

Kiss My Face   Natural Mascara
NaturElle   Ellegance Mascara
                        Ellegance Performance Mascara
Paul Penders   Nutritious Color Mascara*
Perfectly Beautiful   Mascara*
Real Purity   Mascara*

Lip Pencils/Liners

Manufacturer	Product
Burt's Bees	Wings of Love Lip Pencils*
Gabriel	Lipliner
NaturElle	Lip Pencils

Lipstick

Manufacturer	Product
Aubrey Organics	Natural Lips*
Burt's Bees	Wings of Love Lipstick*
Dr. Hauschka	Lip Color*
Gabriel	Lipstick
Kiss My Face	Natural Lipsticks
NaturElle	Premiere Lipstick
Real Purity	Lipstick*

Lip Balms/Gloss

Manufacturer	Product
Burt's Bees	Farmer's Market Lip Gloss*
	Wings of Love Lip Shimmers*
Dr. Hauschka	Lip Balm*
	Lip Care Stick*
Gabriel	Gloss Treatment
Jakaré	Lip Protecting Treatment
Two Star Dog	Lip Balm

Part III	Building a
❧	Beautiful Life

10

Beauty from the Inside Out

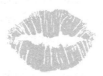

"Take care of your body with steadfast fidelity."
—Johann Wolfgang von Goethe

Creating beauty that lasts a lifetime requires more than stocking your bathroom with natural cosmetics and personal care products. Without the underpinnings of true health, your outward appearance is just window dressing. A smart diet, healthy exercise, and proper rest can make the difference between looks that begin to wane when you hit age thirty and vibrant beauty that can last well into your fifties, sixties, and beyond.

Reducing Your Toxic Burden

Living in a toxic world can make it difficult to achieve true health. Industrial chemicals as well as air and water pollution pose constant threats. Notwithstanding, the personal choices we make every day may have an even bigger impact on our health. Sugar, caffeine, recreational and prescription drugs, alcohol, and nicotine can be the icing on the toxic cake leading to our demise.

Before you can begin your journey toward healthful beauty, it's necessary to break the unhealthy habits that control your life. One way to gain control over these bad habits and speed the removal of toxins from your body is through detoxing. The methods described in this section for banishing accumulated toxins from your body are both effective and easy to do.

Fasting is the quickest way to detoxify your body. Fasting will flush toxins out of your system with amazing speed and allow your body to rest and repair itself. While a strict water fast may be too much for most people, a fast based on freshly squeezed fruit and vegetable juices is a pleasant way to give your body a break, leaving you with increased energy and a greater commitment to healthy living.

A juice fast can last a day or extend up to a full week. To get the maximum benefits from your fast, choose only freshly squeezed juice from organic fruits and vegetables. Canned and bottled varieties often contain pesticide residues and lack the high-quality vitamin and mineral content of fresh produce. Apple juice, spiked with a bit of lemon, or plain carrot juice is basic to any juice fast, but beets, parsley, spinach, cucumber, zucchini, celery, and cabbage are all nutrient-rich choices. For variety, try different combinations of several fruits or vegetables.

A more substantial form of fasting is the mono-food detox method. Instead of consumption of juices, this fast limits you to brown rice and water. Although this form of cleansing isn't a fast in the true sense of the word, it will help detoxify your body and leave you feeling lighter and more energetic. Simply pick a day, and limit yourself to plain brown rice cooked with a bit of sea salt or naturally fermented soy sauce. Make sure you drink eight 8-ounce glasses of water throughout the day to help your body process the rice.

If you prefer a less radical approach to cleansing, consider an herbal detox. Herbs have been used for centuries to accelerate internal cleansing and healing. In fact, among the oldest methods of detoxing in human history, the use of herbs is second only to fasting. While many herbs have been used with success, the most effective cleansing herb is milk thistle, often called the "liver-loving" herb.

Why is the liver so important? The liver prevents toxins from overwhelming the body by breaking them down into less harmful compounds that are eventually flushed out of our system. A constant barrage of toxins can overburden the liver and result in damage. Fortunately, milk thistle strengthens the liver and reduces the damage from the toxins we encounter.

Milk thistle's key component is a bioflavonoid complex known as silymarin. A potent antioxidant and intermediate in cell metabolism, silymarin specifically targets the liver, preventing the depletion of glutathione. Glutathione is a powerful antitoxin that protects the body from environmental and metabolic toxins. Several studies conducted by the Center for Cancer

Causation and Prevention at Denver's AMC Cancer Research Center have also found that milk thistle provides protection against carcinogens. Tests of milk thistle's impact on carcinogenic prostate, breast, and cervical cells showed a significant inhibition of these cancer cells.[1] Better yet, studies demonstrate that milk thistle helps the liver replace dead or damaged cells with healthy new cells, effectively helping the organ repair itself.

Two herbs that play a supporting role in liver health are dandelion and artichoke leaf. Packed with flavonoids, dandelion supports the liver in eliminating toxins and acts as a blood cleanser. It also functions as a diuretic, helping to flush toxins out of the system. Artichoke leaf is also rich in flavonoids and polyphenols, which help heal a compromised liver.[2]

Other herbs work to detoxify the blood, kidneys, and lymphatic system. Garlic, red clover, burdock root, and yellow dock are wonderful blood cleansers. Echinacea and mullein can help detoxify the lymphatic system. And parsley flushes toxins out of the kidneys.

Detoxing with herbs can take several weeks, and you won't experience the dramatic physical changes that accompany a fast. However, if you combine this method with the health-supporting activities described in the following sections, you will notice subtle changes in how you feel and look. Although you can prepare herbal teas or take the individual supplements of each of these herbs, a more convenient way to detox is with one of the commercial cleansing formulas available in most health food stores. One of the best on the market is Zand's Thistle Cleanse, which combines milk thistle, dandelion, yellow dock, red clover, burdock, and licorice with other health-supporting herbs.

Whichever type of cleansing regime you choose, try to detox at least once every three months. An excellent time is at the beginning of each new season. Once you've experienced the benefits of detoxification, you'll wonder how you ever survived without it!

Yes, You Really Are What You Eat

In a world of fast food, desk jobs, and remote controls, it's no surprise that most of us are carrying around more weight than we should. The sad fact is that more than 35 million people in the United States are obese—a statistic that has resulted in a sharp rise in heart disease, diabetes, cancer, and other food-related health problems.

The human body is designed to use food as fuel for energy and as raw material to repair itself. Unfortunately, our eating habits frequently undermine nature's plan. Breakfast is something in which we might indulge—if we have time. Lunch is usually a quick stop for a Big Mac. When it comes to dinner, we often put convenience ahead of nutrition, grabbing whatever is quick and easy. In between, we graze, we nibble, we snack—often out of obsession instead of real hunger.

While our diets are deeply rooted in habit—we prefer eating the familiar foods with which we grew up—cultural pressure plays a part too. Beginning in early childhood, we are conditioned to be members of the "clean-plate club." Because we have fond memories of the sweet treats that followed childhood meals, we reward ourselves with our favorite goodies at every opportunity. We eat when we're stressed or depressed. We even use food as a cure for boredom. The constant barrage of advertisements for snack and convenience foods simply reinforces these patterns. To make matters worse, we let ourselves get caught up in the fast pace of everyday living, often allowing ourselves only enough time to satisfy hunger, not thinking about what we are eating or how it affects our health and our looks.

Centuries ago, Japanese women made the first connection between beauty and nutrition, believing that eating kelp and seafood contributed to sleek, glossy hair. As a bonus, they discovered that their low-fat, low-protein diet of rice and vegetables helped keep them slim and energetic. Today's experts agree that a diet high in fruits and vegetables and low in saturated fat, sugar, and processed or refined foods benefits not only your health but also your looks.

One way to ensure you are getting the nutrition you need is to build your diet around whole foods. Reduce the amount of processed food you consume, and lean toward a more vegetarian diet. The following food plan, created by the Physicians Committee for Responsible Medicine, radically revises the four food groups and can give you a starting point for healthy eating:[3]

1. Whole grains such as brown rice, whole-grain breads, cereals, and pasta: five or more servings a day
2. Legumes such as beans and peas: two to three servings a day
3. Vegetables, raw or lightly cooked: three or more servings a day
4. Fruits: three or more servings a day

You'll notice that meat, eggs, and dairy products aren't included in the new food groups. Although we've been taught to believe that we need lots of animal-based protein to keep us strong, the Physicians Committee for Responsible Medicine considers these foods optional. Nutrition experts are discovering that eating too much protein can be one of the worst culprits undermining our quest for good nutrition.

How much protein do we really need? The average American consumes 90 to 120 grams of protein a day.[4] Yet, according to the World Health Organization, protein should make up only 8 percent of our total diet.[5] That translates to a mere 20 to 40 grams of protein a day—news the beef and dairy industries don't want you to hear. What's more, recent research has linked high levels of dietary protein, especially from animal sources, to osteoporosis and breast cancer.

Another detriment to a healthy diet is fat. Although certain fats and oils are essential for healthy, attractive skin, too much of the wrong fats and oils can wreak havoc with our health and our complexions. Speaking strictly in terms of our looks, an overabundance of saturated fat causes our sebaceous glands to go into overdrive, producing more oil than our systems can handle. Breakouts are often the result. Dr. Elson Haas suggests avoiding the saturated fats contained in animal products, as well as fried foods and the hydrogenated oils used in margarine, baked goods, and many commercially prepared junk foods.[6]

While we consume far too much fat in our diets, there are certain fats that our bodies need. Essential fatty acids (EFAs), commonly referred to as omega-3 and omega-6, are necessary to rebuild and produce new cells. Along with reducing the risk of heart disease and lowering cholesterol, EFAs improve hair, skin, and nails. Good sources of omega-3 EFAs include deepwater fish such as salmon, flaxseeds, and some vegetable oils such as canola and walnut oil. Omega-6 EFAs can be found in raw nuts, seeds, and beans. Performing double duty, soy-based products are an excellent source of both omega-3 and omega-6 EFAs.

Fiber is another key component of a healthy diet. Dietary fiber helps keep the colon clean and prevents the buildup of toxins in the body, which can lead to disease, not to mention skin problems. Fiber-rich beans and peas, whole-grain breads and cereals, and raw fruits and vegetables all contribute to a smart diet.

What about vitamins? Vitamins have become the latest buzzword in the cosmetics industry, with manufacturers scrambling to include nourishing (but often synthetic) nutrients, such as vitamin E, in their products. But despite the claims made by cosmetics companies, there isn't a cosmetic in the world that can take the place of good nutrition. When it comes to healthy looks, here are the most important nutrients in your diet:

- Vitamin A, which you get from broccoli, carrots, spinach, cantaloupe, and peaches, preserves elasticity and helps the skin resist infection and blemishes.
- B complex vitamins, present in whole grains and legumes, are essential for smooth skin, helping to reduce oiliness and the formation of blackheads.
- Vitamin C is an antioxidant required for tissue growth and repair. Essential to the production of collagen, vitamin C also protects the skin from the harmful effects of pollution. Berries, citrus fruits, and green vegetables are all excellent sources of vitamin C.
- Vitamin E, another antioxidant that promotes tissue repair and improves circulation, benefits both skin and hair. Sources include brown rice, soybeans, sweet potatoes, and wheat germ.
- Zinc, available from legumes, mushrooms, soy products, and whole grains, regulates the activity of oil glands and may help prevent acne. It's also required in the formation of collagen and promotes more efficient healing of skin infections.

There's no trick to maintaining a healthy diet. By adhering to these simple guidelines, you can nourish your body beautifully and attain your natural body weight without deprivation or "crash diets":

- **Listen to your body.** Your body is unique, and so are its needs. The best food choices for one person are not necessarily the optimum foods for another. Learn to listen to your body's signs and sensations. It will take some practice, but in time your body will let you know which foods are right for you.

- **Know what's in your food.** Are you getting more than you pay for at the supermarket? The Environmental Protection Agency has identified meat and dairy products as a source of dioxin exposure.[7] Pesticide residue can be detected on most supermarket produce, especially imported varieties, and chemical additives are often included in packaged foods to enhance flavor or prevent spoilage. In fact, the packaging itself can transfer hormone-disrupting phthalates from the plastic into the food.

Of course, it may not always be easy to identify an adulterated food, particularly if it has been genetically modified. Genetically modified foods contain genes that are not naturally found in them. These crops are engineered in a laboratory to alter their genetic blueprint. Soybeans, corn, canola, potatoes, tomatoes, peppers, squash, and dairy products are among the foods most often modified.[8] Genetically engineered foods have been dubbed "frankenfoods" by critics, and the long-term safety of consumption has not been established. How can you tell if a food has been genetically engineered? You can't. Despite a growing consumer movement to label genetically modified food, no laws currently exist that require producers to do so.

• **Go organic.** Don't make dinnertime a toxic experience. Eat organic foods as often as possible. Organic foods offer a safe and sustainable food supply. Moreover, researchers are finding evidence that organically grown produce contains more nutrients than conventionally grown plants.[9] But it isn't so much what you get when you eat organic foods, as what you don't. Organic foods are free of pesticide and herbicide residue, free of growth hormones, and not genetically altered. Health food stores are good places to shop for organic foods, and certified organic produce is beginning to make an appearance in some major grocery stores.

• **Cut down on animal foods, or omit them entirely.** Limiting your consumption of meat and dairy products helps you avoid overdosing on protein and the saturated fats in meats, cheeses, and milk. By eating lower on the food chain (using the new four food groups to guide you), you'll also be consuming fewer pesticides and additives.

• **Don't eat unless you are hungry.** Eating for the wrong reasons increases our consumption of junk food along with our weight.

• **Drink lots of water.** You've heard it before, but it bears repeating. Drink at least eight 8-ounce glasses a day to flush toxins and impurities out of your system. As Dr. Haas likes to say, "Dilution is the solution to [internal] pollution."[10] Unless you have a purification system, don't drink tap water. Opt for bottled purified or distilled water instead.

How we eat is just as important to our health as what we put into our bodies. Eating should be a joyful, nourishing experience. As M. F. K. Fisher said, "Any time we eat it's holy. We should have ritual and ceremony, not just gobbling down some food to keep alive." Deliberate and thoughtful eating connects you with your physical, emotional, and spiritual self. Sit down, turn off the TV, and eat in silence, focusing only on the food in front of you. Giving your undivided attention to a good meal can nourish your senses as well as your body. Appreciating the variety of tastes, colors, and textures can make even the simplest meal special. Savor each bite with your entire being. Enjoy!

Move Gently into the Day

Exercise is an essential component of good health and beauty. A good workout can burn calories, release toxins from your system, keep your muscles toned and flexible, stimulate mental clarity, and increase your energy level. It also promotes the production of endorphins, the body's own natural "feelgood" drug. So, why do we hate to do it? During the 1980s and early 1990s, fitness gurus, from Jane Fonda to Susan Powter, convinced us that we had to push our bodies to the extreme in the name of fitness.

Luckily, the decades of "no pain, no gain" have given way to a saner exercise regime. While a sedentary lifestyle will inevitably result in poor health and excess weight gain, many experts now agree that overdoing fitness can be just as harmful as not exercising at all. They recommend more sustainable forms of exercise such as walking, yoga, and tai chi. These forms of exercise don't require any special equipment and can be practiced by anyone, regardless of age. So, throw away all those exercise tapes bought in desperation, and let's look at the new way to exercise! Note: Before beginning *any* new exercise routine, discuss the program with your health care practitioner.

Stretching

If you spend a lot of time in sedentary activities, you may be disappointed to discover that your body doesn't move the way it used to. If the muscles in your body aren't used on a regular basis, they begin to lose tone and function, leaving you stiff and sore. Stretching is a great way to increase and maintain flexibility.

Before you begin, relax your body by shaking out your arms and legs. Using slow movements and rhythmic breathing, stretch each part of your body in turn. Don't jerk or bounce. Incorporating a few minutes of stretching into your daily routine will keep your body fluid and ready to meet the demands of your day.

If simple stretching doesn't provide enough challenge, you may want to explore a more structured routine involving yoga.

Yoga

Yoga originated more than six thousand years ago in India. Founded by Tibetan monks, yoga takes its name from the ancient Sanskrit word meaning to unite or join. A traditional yogi (one who practices yoga) strives to unite the conscious mind with the unconscious or universal mind, ultimately resulting in a totally integrated personality.

Over the past thirty years, the Western world has adopted yoga as a therapeutic form of exercise, with an emphasis on deep breathing, relaxed movements, and mental concentration. Among the many benefits of yoga are increased flexibility, toning and rejuvenating the nervous system, and improved circulation. It also cultivates the shape, grace, and beauty of the body.

Yoga is simply a series of asanas, or poses, which are best learned and practiced under the guidance of a qualified teacher. Although there are well-illustrated and comprehensive books on the subject, it's a difficult art to master from a series of pictures. Yoga centers have been established across the country and offer enjoyable classes suited to all levels of mastery, from beginner to advanced. In addition, classes in yoga are often offered through local community centers or colleges.

Tai Chi

Although tai chi is a centuries-old offshoot of yoga, it departs from the still-life asanas of yoga and embodies the world of moving meditation. The heart of the practice is the Chinese concept of chi (pronounced "chee"), roughly translated to mean the life force or vital energy of the universe. This energy flows through all of nature, including human beings. Based on the movements of animals, tai chi is composed of slow, dancelike steps and gestures. The weight of the body shifts continually from one foot to the other as the movements are performed in a series of circles, arcs, and spirals. The fluidity and grace of this form of exercise encourages relaxation and mental peace, as well as balance and flexibility. A qualified instructor is essential, and classes are offered at many martial arts schools.

Qigong

Qigong is an ancient Taoist system of exercise that complements both yoga and tai chi. Healing qigong combines breath work, gentle movements, and meditative postures to harmonize the body, mind, and spirit. Because of its positive effect on strength, stamina, flexibility, posture, and concentration, the practice of qigong will enhance your physical performance, improve sleep, help balance stress, boost energy levels, and clarify your mind. Unfortunately, there aren't many qigong classes available at this time, but it is easy to learn, and there are some excellent videos on the market.

Walking

If your cardiovascular system needs a workout, go for a walk! Walking is one of the best aerobic exercises around. Providing a complete workout, walking doesn't require any special equipment and carries the least risk of injury of any form of exercise. Best of all, you can do it anywhere, whether you live in the city, the country, or somewhere in between.

If you're not used to exercising, start slowly, limiting yourself to a ten-minute walk. As your stamina increases, you should be able to gradually increase your trek to forty-five minutes. Although walking is something you've done all your life, there are a few things to keep in mind in order to do it right. First, find a pair of comfortable walking shoes—nothing undermines your daily walk faster then a painful blister or two. Walk briskly, and practice good posture. Develop a good breathing pattern, and keep your body aligned and relaxed. Finally, walk every day. If inclement weather threatens your plans, try doing a few laps through a shopping mall (minus the pit stops at your favorite stores), or use a treadmill if you have access to one.

Weight Training

Weight training is another low-impact way to a fit life, particularly when it's combined with walking. Not only will weight training help strengthen your muscles and sculpt your body, but it can actually help build your bones as well. According to the National Institutes of Health Osteoporosis and Related Bone Diseases National Resource Center, 8 million American women suffer from osteoporosis, and millions more have low bone mass.[11] Although walking and other weight-bearing exercise programs are recognized as one of the ways to prevent bone loss, researchers at the University of California, Los Angeles, say it may not be enough. They speculate that walking combined with resistance-type exercise such as weight training not only helps prevent bone loss but also may actually enhance bone mineralization.[12]

Many health clubs, colleges, and recreation centers are equipped with weight machines that can provide the resistance necessary to benefit bones. But before you begin, make sure you get instruction on the proper way to use the machines. To prevent sore muscles and possible injury, it's wise to start slowly. Set the machine at the lowest weight possible, and start by doing eight to ten repetitions on each. Over the next few weeks, increase the weight and the number of repetitions. Although committing to a regular weight-training routine—at least three times a week—may require a bit of willpower, the rewards are priceless: beautiful bones and a stronger, leaner body.

Sleeping Beauty

Waking up from a night's rest should leave you feeling refreshed and alive, ready to meet the new day. A good night's sleep is essential for us to look and feel our best, but too often we shortchange ourselves in the amount of sleep we actually need. While an occasional late night won't do any lasting harm, sleeping poorly or getting into the habit of too little sleep can result in dark circles, sallow skin, poor concentration, and eventually illness.

As difficult as it may seem in our nonstop schedules, it's important to block out enough time for your body to rejuvenate itself. Although eight hours is the traditional amount of sleep necessary to maintain good health, you may need more or less than the standard eight hours. Experiment and see what works for you.

What about those nights when you toss and turn, thoughts racing through your mind? Nights when every noise rankles and every ache or pain is amplified? We all have times when sleep seems to elude us. Here are a few suggestions to help you relax:

- Try to get to bed by 10:00 P.M. This helps regulate and align your body to its natural sleep cycle.
- If noise is a problem, invest in a white noise or sound machine, or play tapes of soft, soothing music and nature sounds to mask offensive noises.
- Your bedroom should be dark, quiet, and used only for sleep. Don't prop yourself up in bed to read, work, or watch TV. Stimulating your mind right before nodding off can result in a poor night's sleep.
- Speaking of stimulation, don't consume caffeine after 7:00 P.M. If you are particularly sensitive to the effects of caffeine, you may want to consider giving it up altogether.
- If you just can't leave the day's activities behind, do a little breath work (you'll learn more about this in the next chapter). Focusing your entire consciousness on your breath makes it difficult for other thoughts to take possession of your mind. After a few minutes of this, you should find that your mind and body have relaxed enough for you to get to sleep. To encourage relaxation, sprinkle a few drops of lavender essential oil on your pillow.
- Stay away from prescription or over-the-counter sleep aids, which can be addictive. For those rare nights when you're plagued by insomnia, try a glass of warm milk. Ayurvedic practitioners suggest adding a pinch of cardamom or nutmeg to enhance the milk's sleep-inducing qualities. For hard-core insomnia, you may want to try kava-kava or valerian, herbal sleep and relaxation aids that have been used for centuries. Although these herbs don't have any side effects and aren't habit-forming, don't become dependent on their use for chronic insomnia.

Body Love

When you were a small child, your body was a celebration. You explored every part of yourself, reveling in the feats your body could perform. You moved gracefully, your limbs and torso in perfect harmony. Your imagination ran wild, and your senses exploded in a rainbow of experiences as you joyfully discovered the world for the first time.

But that was then, and this is now. The older we get, the more divorced we become from the natural comfort we once had with our bodies, becoming caught up in the religious and moral taboos that surround our physical selves. We are quickly taught which parts of our body are acceptable and which are not. When we were in school, our teachers gave precedence to the mind, stressing logic and knowledge as the ultimate goal. However, while logic helps us develop common sense and knowledge should be a lifelong quest, they're only part of the human experience. To be truly integrated, we must also nurture our physical selves.

Poor body image is another deterrent. Continually inundated by the media, we constantly compare our own bodies with the "perfect" women we see on television and in magazines. Regardless of the fact that this "Barbie doll" ideal doesn't reflect reality, we reject and rebel against our own bodies, perceiving faults that may or may not be real—our legs are too short, our eyes are too close together, our breasts are too big or small, we're too fat, we're too thin. From puberty onward, we spend our lives remodeling our physical selves, often enduring an endless series of crash diets and fad exercise programs. Some of us become so obsessed with our image that we willingly succumb to plastic surgery, dangerous weight-loss drugs, and even eating disorders. It's a vicious cycle leading to low self-esteem and, for some, life-threatening health problems.

Learning to free yourself from "imageitis" isn't easy. Often, it's hard to look at your body and see a unique, beautiful, and sexual being. Yet, you are. To fight a lifetime of conditioning requires us to radically change the way we think of our bodies. We need to remodel not our bodies, but our minds.

The next time you pass a mirror, pause and look at your reflection. Tell yourself, out loud if you are alone, that you're the most beautiful woman ever born. It doesn't matter if you've just gotten out of bed or if you're dressed to the nines. Just say it! Practice this simple exercise every time you're in the vicinity of a mirror. You may feel a bit foolish at first, but each time you do this simple exercise, you're teaching yourself to view your body differently, removing another chunk of the media's stereotype to reveal the real woman beneath. In time, you'll begin to believe the words and realize how special you really are.

Body gazing is another way to overcome the negative image we have of our physical selves. To begin, choose some time when you are alone. Soften the lights, and stand naked in front of a full-length mirror. Although gazing at your body may make you feel odd or self-conscious at first, bringing up old taboos and feelings of guilt, remember that your body is a temple and was, at one time in your life, a source of wonder and pleasure. Your body tells your life story, an expression of all your thoughts and feelings. By forming a positive relationship with your body, you become more accepting of every aspect of yourself.

Through the ages, the concepts of beauty and femininity were firmly rooted in a woman's unique role as nurturer and life giver. Ancient carvings of Venus, the mythical goddess of sexuality and desire, show a figure with full breasts, an ample belly, and lush, wide hips. The most beautiful nudes ever painted were by Rubens and Raphael and depicted the ideal woman as plump and curvaceous. Even today, large, well-seasoned women are revered among many third-world cultures, bringing forth visions of the earth mother. Over the centuries, this well-endowed figure has evoked not only respect but passion. As late as the 1950s, the full-bodied curves of Marilyn Monroe, poured into her size 16 dresses, held the world entranced. These are the images we must carry with us as we practice body gazing.

Close your eyes and take a few minutes to consider your body in an uncritical manner. It is unique, like no other. It is a reflection of divine energy and is sacred. Now open your eyes. Begin with the top of your head and slowly look at each part of your body. Do this without rejecting any part of yourself.

If you still can't get past the Madison Avenue hype, try thinking of the wonderful contribution each part of your body makes to your life. Your face is the canvas on which your emotions are painted and gives the world a glimpse of who you are. Each scar and wrinkle tells a tale. Your arms comfort and express your love with their embraces. Connecting us to others are our hands, giving us the power to touch, heal, and create. No matter their size or shape, your breasts contain the capacity for pleasure and nourishment. Your belly is the center of your being. Like the fertile earth that brings forth life, your belly is the origin of humanity. Your hips are the cradle for this miracle of birth. Supporting your entire being, your legs and feet ground you to the earth and all life.

Using these different mental images as we look upon our bodies, we begin to see our bodies as the rich, vibrant expression of womanhood valued through the ages. In the postindustrialized West, women have been denied this legacy, bound instead to a thin, perpetually childlike image disconnected from nature.

Self-massage is another wonderful way to become comfortable and connected with your body. It's typical to touch ourselves only when we are in pain or discomfort. Through self-massage, you become intimately aware of the various sensations your body experiences.

To give yourself a massage, sit or lie in a comfortable position with your eyes closed. Take several slow, deep breaths to relax yourself, and let your hands drift to any part of the body they desire. There's no set pattern to follow. You may limit yourself to selected areas of your body or explore it in its entirety. Working slowly and rhythmically, gently stroke and caress whichever part of your body you wish. Focus your entire awareness on the sensations you feel. The more often you give yourself a massage, the more comfortable you'll become with your physical self.

For variety, use a fragrant body lotion or massage oil for a whole-body massage, beginning with your forehead and ending with your toes. By experiencing your entire body, you bring a sense of connection and wholeness to your inner and outer self.

By routinely assessing yourself in new, more loving ways, you begin the gradual process of accepting your body as it is. As we learn to accept, appreciate, and love our own bodies, we discover this attitude spilling over into other areas of our lives. Our self-confidence increases, giving us the courage to explore the unknown. We become less fearful of growing older and find ourselves deliberately taking time to celebrate our bodies and our lives.

11

Discovering Your Beautiful Spirit

"Women who live for the next miracle cream do not realize that beauty comes from a secret happiness and equilibrium within themselves."

—Sophia Loren

Given enough money, anyone can buy superficial beauty. Synthetic paints and powders, not to mention cosmetic surgery, can produce any look we want. But it is just a facade and doesn't reflect who we really are. Without a deeper wholeness, superficial beauty is like the image in a mirror, lacking substance and life. If you throw something at it, the image shatters.

Inner harmony is the piece that completes the picture of true, lasting beauty. Spiritual grounding and a strong sense of self, combined with a luscious enthusiasm for life, can make any woman irresistible. Consciously nurturing your whole self is the first step on a journey toward revealing the real beauty you possess.

Decompress Stress

One of the worst toxins with which we come in contact every day isn't created in a lab or sold in stores. It's stress. In fact, it's estimated that 75 percent of all visits to the doctor's office are due to stress-related ailments.[1]

Stress is a pervasive factor of modern life, making us feel insecure and overwhelmed. We worry about our families, our health, how we're going to pay the bills, and whether or not we'll still have a job tomorrow. Escalating crime and environmental problems press in around us, leaving us wondering if we'll be the next to fall victim in a world that seems out of control. Living with these concerns day in and day out, we bury our stress, masking it with increased activity.

As our days become filled with "essential" commitments, we set aside our dreams and desires, allowing ourselves to be buried under an avalanche of never-ending "shoulds." We've become so overcommitted that some days, it's hard just to keep up. We're left with the uneasy feeling that we're not really in control of our lives. We're anxious and isolated, living a life without joy. The Hopi Indians have a name for it—*koyanisquatsi*, or "life out of balance."

Although society puts an enormous amount of pressure on us to perform, it's our own unrealistic expectations that cause the most stress in our lives—to be the perfect employee, the perfect lover, the perfect parent, the perfect friend—expectations that prevent us from owning our lives.

Allowing ourselves to become overly stressed in the quest to meet these superhuman demands is often a sign that we've stopped paying attention to who we really are. American writer and Trappist monk Thomas Merton once asked, "What can we gain by sailing to the moon if we are not able to cross the abyss that separates us from ourselves?" Ignoring our own needs restricts our potential for personal growth, damages our self-esteem, and limits our capacity to become happier, more fulfilled human beings.

Stress also has a direct effect on our looks. Besides making us look and feel frazzled, stress depletes our bodies of vitamins A, C, and E, as well as the B complex nutrients needed for strong hair, skin, and nails. Prolonged stress can wreak havoc with the adrenal glands, resulting in an increase of cortisol and the male hormone androgen. Too much androgen can cause hair to become brittle and increases sebum production, ultimately leading to clogged pores and blemishes.

Although it's difficult to disengage from the demands of everyday life, learning to relax is essential to our looks, our health, and our well-being. We can no longer consider "downtime" a luxury. What can we do to diminish the stress in our lives and truly care for ourselves? Here are a few ways to dispel the constant tension that overwhelms us, nourish our inner selves, and, in the process, rediscover the beautiful odyssey called life.

Give Yourself a Break

Clearing stress from our lives may free our minds and bolster our health, but embracing a more relaxed way of living doesn't happen overnight. Instead of striving to be perfect, embrace imperfection. Impossible as it may seem, the world won't end if you don't get every single thing on your "to do" list accomplished. Learn to set priorities. Break tasks down into three categories—critical, important, and nonessential—and then throw out all the nonessential tasks. Concentrate on the critical chores, and then work on as many of the important tasks as you can comfortably fit into your day.

Another way to reduce your "to do" list is by learning to delegate. It may sound simple, but asking for help from a mate, coworkers, or children takes practice and patience. It's often difficult to hand responsibility over to others because we falsely equate asking for help with being weak and dependent. Remember that, along with lightening your own load, sharing responsibility for everyday tasks can give others the opportunity to develop skills and build self-esteem.

Laugh a Lot

Laughter is good for the soul, and recent studies indicate that using a little jocularity to manage stress can help keep you healthy. "Stress sets off a number of negative reactions," says Steve Allen Jr., M.D., clinical assistant professor at New York's State University and son of the famous comedian. "Aside from lowering our overall resistance to illness, research has shown that stress causes an overdose of adrenaline and cortisone in our systems, as well as the production of stomach acid. Luckily, laughter increases the body's tolerance to these negative chemical effects."[2] Recent studies have also demonstrated that laughter plays a role in reducing pain, improving immunity, and lowering blood pressure.[3]

Besides keeping us physically and mentally balanced, humor can make us feel in charge of our lives. Joel Goodman, Ph.D., director of The Humor Project, Inc., calls humor "power." According to Goodman, "You can't always control situations around you, but you can control your internal responses to them with humor. That's power."[4]

Learning to laugh at ourselves is one of the best ways to reduce the amount of pressure we put on ourselves to be perfect. Spend five or ten minutes a day looking for the funny side of life. Create a humor bulletin board at home or at work. Tack up cartoons and jokes that make you chuckle, funny photos, or special mementos that make you smile. Collect silly things that make you laugh—children's toys, clown noses, funny hats—and play with them often. Dr. Allen, who practices juggling in his office (much to the delight of himself and his patients), points out that the true meaning of the word *silly* is to be blessed, prosperous, happy, and healthy.

Dance in the Rain

Ignoring our need for relaxation and joyful play limits our capacity to become happier, more fulfilled human beings. Being a responsible grown-up all day, every day restricts our growth and our ability to trust our intuition. In fact, many therapists and researchers believe that society's overwhelming sense of urgency and speed, combined with our own unrealistic expectations, results in a loss of connection to the soul, to the child we once were.

Play takes us out of our everyday world, transporting us back to the freedom of childhood. We find ourselves in a place where it's OK to act silly, get dirty, and be outrageous. Suddenly, we become aware that play is psychically reintegrating, adding a higher level of meaning to our lives. Creating moments of joy in our lives helps us to reconnect to who we really are. It keeps us from taking ourselves too seriously and recharges our spirit, helping us to better cope with all the "shoulds" in our lives. It's during these moments of pleasure that we feel most alive.

The next time you feel frantic and overwhelmed by the pressures of adulthood—play! Dance, skip, run . . . just for the sheer joy of it. Walk in the rain and let your inhibitions melt away. Smell the fragrance of the world being washed new. Find the biggest puddle *and jump in*! Borrow from your childhood. Make a finger painting, pick wildflowers, or sing as loudly as you can! Whatever you choose to do, let it bring you into the moment.

As you become more comfortable indulging in playful moments, you'll find that play isn't so much a time-consuming activity as it is a state of mind. It may not take any more time to approach life with a playful attitude, but it will make a difference in how you feel about yourself and your life at the end of the day.

Slow Down

Instead of mindlessly zipping through the tasks of the day, slow down! Slowing down the pace of our lives gives us the sense of living deliberately, of being in charge of our lives. It gives us time to evaluate our life situations, to listen to our instincts, and to wisely choose how we really want to live.

If slowing down seems impossible, start with the small tasks you do every day. Hang the laundry out in the sun instead of tossing it in the dryer. Wash the dishes by hand. Try walking instead of riding. Before you begin an activity, consciously think of ways to do it slowly. Taking the hustle and bustle out of life's little chores gives your mind a chance to settle, making it easier to connect with your inner self.

Quiet Your Mind

It's difficult to relax when your mind is constantly chattering. Tasks, large and small, compete for your attention. Regrets from the past and plans for the future bounce into and out of your mind with amazing speed. It's as though a half dozen monkeys are cavorting in your head, each with its own agenda and all of them pulling in different directions. One of the easiest ways to calm this circus of thought is to practice breath focus. Turning all of your attention to the physical act of breathing brings you into the present moment and leaves no room for thoughts of the past or future . . . there is only the *now*.

Breath work can be practiced anytime you feel tense or overwhelmed. Even a few minutes of breath focus can calm and quiet your mind, leaving you feeling refreshed and tranquil. It's especially useful just before falling asleep.

To begin, close your eyes and breathe normally. Take a slow, deep breath through your nose. Note how your lungs expand as your diaphragm rises. Imagine that you are filling your whole body with calming energy. Now exhale through your mouth, releasing all of the built-up stress within you. Silently repeat the following words as you practice: *In* . . . you know you are breathing in; *Out* . . . you know you are breathing out; *Calm* . . . the calming energy of the universe is flowing through you; *Release* . . . you are releasing the tension from your mind and body.

Create a Sanctuary

Wouldn't it be lovely if we could each have a room of our very own, a place where we could shut out the demands of the day and hide for a while. While having a room of our own may not be practical for most of us, we can find some private space in our lives where we can slow down and become centered.

It may be a chair in the corner, a fragrant bath, or a quiet spot in the garden—anywhere that provides you with stillness and solitude.

Think of your sanctuary as a miniretreat, a haven where you can be alone with your thoughts and put the day into perspective. Turn off the tube and unplug the phone. Don't allow intruders to break into your peace. Create an atmosphere of tranquility, nurturing your senses with fragrant candles or essential oil. Turn on some soothing music. The important thing is to find a place that's yours and yours alone. A place where you can spend quiet time regaining your balance when life throws you off track.

Empower Yourself

We all know someone who radiates a special beauty that can't be obtained from any cosmetics. No matter what the person's outward appearance, we are naturally drawn to the altruistic nature and sense of self-confidence. What is it that sets such people apart? They are empowered by a deeper knowledge of themselves and their role in the human drama we call life.

Reaching inward to unearth your own beautiful spirit is a rewarding but solitary journey. The answers you'll discover along the way can't be found in any book or self-improvement program. There are no steps to follow, nor any map to lead you on your way. There are, however, tools you can use to help you discover your personal power.

Tap into Your Creativity

We are all born with the capacity to be creative. Unfortunately, as we grow up, our creative side is often criticized, stifled, or undervalued. The result can be an uninspired life, devoid of outlets for creativity and imagination.

The good news is that the creativity of your childhood still lurks deep within you. All it takes is a little coaxing to bring your artistic side to the surface. In her book *The Artist's Way*, Julia Cameron suggests making a "date" with your inner artist, scheduling regular blocks of time to nurture your creative consciousness.[5] Paint a picture. Write a poem. Cook a fabulous meal. Decorate a room.

It doesn't matter what the end result is, as long as you pour your heart into it. Talent is not the issue here. The point is to create for the sheer joy of creating.

Nurturing our creativity also helps us develop a sense of *being*—and allows us to grow inwardly and outwardly.[6] When you give yourself permission to be creative, you will find that, along with freeing yourself from stress, expanding your artistic side also frees your soul.

Start a Journal

Keeping a journal can help you resolve conflicts, release bottled-up emotions, and deal with life's disappointments. It's a private place where you can drop the mask of civility and let off steam. Keeping a journal is a remarkably effective way to help balance your emotional and mental well-being. It can help you decide what's really important in your life and what you can release. It can also help you uncover the truths that have been buried under years of denial—denial that can impede your journey and keep you from realizing your full potential.

A good way to begin is to write about the most stressful event in your life. Don't worry about grammar or spelling—simply write. Write nonstop—give vent to all of the emotions surrounding the event—but don't limit yourself to your emotions. Make sure you include the facts surrounding the event. By writing about what happened *and* how it makes you feel, you'll have a better grasp of both the experience and your reaction to it. As an old Chinese proverb says, "Hearing, I forget. Seeing, I remember. Writing, I understand."

Although there are beautiful journals on the market that you can use, yours can be as simple as a spiral-bound notebook or a legal pad. Whatever type of journal you decide to keep, write often and on a regular basis. Liberating ourselves from deep-seated beliefs and behavioral patterns can't be accomplished on a hit-or-miss basis.

At times, you may find that writing in your journal is a painful experience, conjuring up feelings of deep sadness, fear, and even panic. Remember, you're touching emotions below the surface in order to heal the emotional upset. Just as curing a physical ailment can sometimes be unpleasant, we may have to work our way through some painful emotions before we can gain insight, acceptance, and finally, resolution.

Meditate

Learning to meditate can also take us beyond the superficiality of everyday life. As more and more people discover the benefits of meditation, the old counterculture image of navel-gazing gurus in a cloud of incense is being replaced by mainstream portraits of executives, athletes, and housewives, all engaging in this 2,500-year-old spiritual practice.

When practiced regularly, meditation can bring a profound sense of mental and physical calm. It opens up a deeper understanding of ourselves and the world around us. Meditation alters our consciousness and helps us to think outside the box.[7] It's not an escape from reality, but a state of mind in which the worry, anger, guilt, and desires that lurk just below the surface of our consciousness can be acknowledged in a nonjudgmental environment.

Meditation is a highly personal, creative experience that brings us closer to our own truth. Through meditation, we can banish the toxic thoughts and behavior patterns that pollute our inner lives and replace them with a deeper understanding and acceptance of who we really are. There are different schools of meditation, including Zen and transcendental among others, but they all develop mindfulness and mental spaciousness, allowing us to see our true nature by using a focus to quiet the mind.

To practice meditation, sit quietly in a comfortable position. As you did in the breathing exercise, focus all your attention on your breath. It's normal for random thoughts to distract you, especially when you are just beginning to learn how to meditate. Each time you become distracted, take note of the thoughts and images, and then gently bring your attention back to your breathing. After a few minutes, expand your awareness to include any sensations your body feels. Begin with a ten-minute meditation session, increasing the time as your practice evolves.

You may be disappointed if it takes some time before you can get rid of the chatter inside your head. Don't give up or chide yourself for not grasping the practice immediately. A highly active mind may take longer to quiet, but the benefits are well worth it. Just continue to practice daily. Eventually, you will be able to still the mental prattle.

As you develop the mental discipline necessary for meditation, you may want to experiment with other focusing tools. Many people find that using a mantra, a meaningful word or phrase, helps them block out mental chatter. An object, such as a flower or a candle, can also serve as a focusing tool.

If you meditate regularly, over time you will notice some profound changes. You'll feel calmer and more relaxed. Your energy level will increase. You may even find your perspective of the world altered to a deeper awareness and a more patient, loving outlook.

Visualize Your Life

Once you have excavated your hidden dreams and desires, consciously visualizing your life as it *could be* can help you achieve the life you want. Visualization is a form of constructive daydreaming that can alter your subconscious thought pattern and help combat the inner voices that keep you from your dreams.

To begin, imagine yourself as you would like to be. If you would like to become a painter, see yourself painting. If you would like to start your own business, picture yourself in that setting. If you would like to change a negative relationship in your life, create an image of your life without this person. See yourself in the situation you have imagined. How does it make you feel? Now picture the steps required to make the image a reality. Create a complete image of each step; don't leave out any details. Before completing your session, conjure up the first image again and tell yourself, "*This* is who I am."

Practicing visualization at least once each day can help us break unwanted habits, replace the negative beliefs that undermine our lives with more positive ones, and give us the courage to make the changes necessary for happier, more fulfilling lives.

Learn to Take Risks

Being truly alive involves taking chances and exploring unknown territory. Throughout our lives, we are faced with thousands of opportunities to expand our horizons and fulfill our potential. Most of us play it safe, doing what's expected of us and wondering what our lives would have been like if only we had taken the chance and followed our hearts. Think back . . . how often have you regretted not taking some action that may have changed your whole life?

The next time life presents you with an opportunity to seize your dreams, go for it! It can be as mundane as changing jobs or as daring as learning to sky dive. Whatever it is, stop making excuses or blaming other people for not being able to realize your full potential. It can be frightening to try something new, and, yes, you may fail, but you may also find rich and rewarding experiences in the unknown.

Tell Your Own Truth

All of the activities just discussed are simply tools to help you discover who you *really* are. Not who your parents, friends, mate, or coworkers think you are. Not who you've been conditioned to believe you are. But your true self. Through these exercises, we meet ourselves, perhaps for the first time.

There will be times on your journey when an inner crisis or a painful truth tempts you to retreat into the safety of your former life, to curl up in a corner and forget the whole thing. Other times may bring anger and tears. After all, the process of uncovering your authentic self carries a sense of loss as well as gain. You are destroying the illusions that have kept you from discovering your authenticity, and doing so can bring sorrow as well as joy.

There may also be times of bewilderment, when we feel lost, with no idea where this whole process of discovery will lead. Instead of allowing frustration to overwhelm us, we must learn to enjoy the gradual unfolding of self.

As you make your pilgrimage toward your own truth, your own power, you will begin to live your life deliberately and joyfully. As you journey down life's road, those around you will discover that you, too, have begun to radiate an inner beauty that comes from the soul and the power to realize your dreams.

Appendix A: Fight Back!

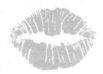

Now that you know the truth about what's really in many of the products you use every day, you can make informed decisions when it's time to go shopping. But simply changing your buying habits will not stop the cosmetics giants from peddling an ever-increasing array of toxic products.

The most effective way to force manufacturers to address the hazards posed by their products is to hit them where it hurts—in their profits. Make your voice heard, and tell the members of the cosmetics industry that you are boycotting their wares until they put women's health first.

The letter included here is just a sample. Feel free to write one that details your specific concerns and experiences.

Sample Boycott Letter

Dear _____:

As a loyal customer, I was appalled to learn how many carcinogens, neurotoxins, and endocrine disruptors are regularly included in your products. These chemicals, mainly petroleum based, may adversely impact my health and the health of millions of American women.

Until your company puts women's health ahead of corporate profit, I will boycott all of your products, relying instead on nontoxic cosmetics and personal care products for my health and beauty needs, and I will encourage my family and friends to do the same.

Sincerely,

[Your Name]

Since corporate America rarely takes action without a regulatory push from the government, you may also want to drop a note to your U.S. senator and/or representative. Check your local telephone book for the address and phone number of your Congressional representatives, or check online at www.congress.org for contact information.

Sample Legislative Letter

Dear _____:

As one of millions of American women who use cosmetics every day, I am very concerned about the health risks that these products pose. Hundreds of synthetic chemicals are routinely included in everything from shampoo to eye shadow, many of which are known carcinogens, neurotoxins, and endocrine disruptors. These substances are a threat not only to human health but to the environment as well. The appalling lack of regulation governing the cosmetics industry prevents the federal Food and Drug Administration from properly protecting consumers from the cumulative long-term dangers of cosmetics use.

On behalf of all women, I hope you will address this issue.

Sincerely,

[Your Name]

Cosmetics Manufacturers Contact Information

Parent Company	Products/Brands
Alberto-Culver Company	Alberto VO-5
2525 Armitage Avenue	FDS
Melrose Park, IL 60160	Just For Me
phone: 708-450-3000	Motions
fax: 708-450-3354	St. Ives Swiss Formula
website: www.alberto.com	Soft and Beautiful
	TCB
	TRESemmé
Avon Products	bath and body care
1345 Avenue of the Americas	color cosmetics
New York, NY 10105	fragrance
phone: 212-282-5000	skin care
fax: 212-282-6056	
website: www.avon.com	
Bath and Body Works	bath and body care
97 W. Main Street	fragrance
New Albany, OH 43054	
phone: 800-395-1001	
fax: 614-856-6818	
website: www.intimatebrands.com	

BeneFit Cosmetics   color cosmetics

685 Market Street   skin care

Seventh Floor

San Francisco, CA 94105

phone: 415-781-8153

fax: 415-781-3930

website: www.benefitcosmetics.com

The Body Shop   bath and body care

5036 One World Way   color cosmetics

Wake Forest, NC 27587   fragrance

phone: 919-544-4900   hair care

fax: 919-544-4361   skin care

website: www.the-body-shop.com

Bonne Bell, Inc.   bath and body care

P.O. Box 770349   color cosmetics

Lakewood, OH 44107   fragrance

phone: 216-221-0800   skin care

fax: 216-221-6256

website: www.bonnebell.com

Chanel, Inc.   color cosmetics

9 W. Fifty-Seventh Street,   fragrance

Forty-Fourth Floor   skin care

New York, NY 10019

phone: 212-688-5055

fax: 212-752-1851

website: www.chanel.com

Christian Dior   color cosmetics

19 E. Fifty-Seventh Street   fragrance

New York, NY   skin care

phone: 212-759-1840

website: www.dior.com

Clarins   fragrance

4, rue Berteaux Dumas   skin care

92203 Neuily-sur Seine, France

phone: +33-1-47-38-12-12

fax: +33-1-47-38-16-87

website: www.clarins.fr

Colgate-Palmolive Company   Lady Speed Stick

300 Park Avenue   Softsoap

New York, NY 10022

phone: 212-310-2000

fax: 212-310-3405

website: www.colgate.com

Combe, Inc.   Grecian 5

1101 Westchester Avenue   Grecian Formula

White Plains, NY 10604   Just 5

phone: 914-694-5454   Just for Men

fax: 914-694-1926

website: www.combe.com

Coty, Inc.

1325 Avenue of the Americas

New York, NY 10019

phone: 212-479-4300

fax: 212-479-4399

website: www.coty.com

Adidas Moves for Her

Casmir

Colour Pure

Davidoff

Exclamation

The Healing Garden

Isabella Rossellini Manifesto

Jil Sander

Joop!

Lancaster

Libertine

Manifesto

Mira Bai

Sensations

Wish

Crabtree and Evelyn, Ltd.

102 Peake Brook Road

Woodstock, CT 06281

phone: 800-272-2873 or 860-928-2761

fax: 860-928-0452

website: www.crabtree-evelyn.com

bath and body care

fragrance

skin care

Del Laboratories, Inc.

178 EAB Plaza

Uniondale, NY 11556

phone: 516-844-2020

fax: 631-293-1515

website: www.dellabs.com

Corn Silk

Naturistics

New York Color

Sally Hansen

Dial Corporation

15501 N. Dial Boulevard

Scottsdale, AZ 85260

phone: 480-754-3425

fax: 480-754-1098

website: www.dialcorp.com

Freeman Cosmetics

Nature's Accents

Sarah Michaels

Elizabeth Arden

14100 N.W. Sixtieth Avenue

Miami Lakes, FL 33014

phone: 305-818-8000

fax: 305-818-8010

website: www.frenchfragrances.com

Calvin Klein

Ceramides

Elizabeth Taylor's White Diamonds

Geoffrey Beene

Giorgio

Halston

Millennium

Nautica

Oscar de la Renta

Passion

Paul Sebastian

Red Door

Visible Difference

Wings

English Ideas, Ltd.   color cosmetics

9251 Irvine Boulevard   skin care

Irvine, CA 92618

phone: 949-789-8790

fax: 949-789-8797

website: www.englishideas.com

Erno Laszlo   color cosmetics

3202 Queens Boulevard   skin care

Long Island City, NY 11101

phone: 718-729-4480

fax: 718-716-3204

website: www.ernolaszlo.com

Estée Lauder Companies   Aveda

767 Fifth Avenue   Bobbi Brown Essentials

New York, NY 10153   Bumble and Bumble

phone: 212-572-4200   Clinique

fax: 212-572-6633   Donna Karan

website: www.elcompanies.com   Estée Lauder

                                        Jane

                                        M.A.C.

                                        Origins

                                        Prescriptives

                                        Tommy

Hard Candy	color cosmetics
661 N. Harper Avenue	nail care
Los Angeles, CA 90048	
phone: 323-658-9099	
fax: 323-658-9093	
website: www.hardcandy.com	

Jafra Cosmetics International	color cosmetics
P.O. Box 5026	skin care
Westlake Village, CA 91359	
phone: 800-551-2345	
fax: 805-449-2909	
website: www.jafra.com	

Johnson and Johnson	Aveeno
1 Johnson and Johnson Plaza	Neutrogena
New Brunswick, NJ 08933	Nizoral
phone: 732-524-0400	RoC
fax: 732-214-0332	Shower to Shower
website: www.jnj.com	T-gel

Johnson Products Company, Inc.	Dermablend
8522 S. Lafayette Avenue	Gentle-Treatment
Chicago, IL 60620	Posner
phone: 800-442-4643 or 773-483-4100	
fax: 773-962-5741	
website: www.sheen.com	

Lamaur Corporation

5601 E. River Road

Minneapolis, MN 55432

phone: 763-571-1234

fax: 763-572-2781

website: www.lamaur.com

Salon Style

Style

Willow Lakes

Lorac Cosmetics, Inc.

9559 Irondale Avenue

Chatsworth, CA 91311

phone: 818-678-3939

fax: 818-678-3930

website: www.loraccosmetics.com

color cosmetics

skin care

L'Oréal S.A.

41 rue Martre

92117 Clichy, France

phone: +33-1-41-56-70-00

fax: +33-1-47-56-80-02

website: www.loreal.com

Biotherm

Giorgio Armani Parfums

Helena Rubinstein

La Roche-Posay

Lancôme Paris

Maybelline

Ralph Lauren Parfums

Redken

Vichy Laboratories

Mary Kay, Inc.	color cosmetics
16251 Dallas Parkway	skin care
Addison, TX 75001	
phone: 972-687-6300	
fax: 972-687-1609	
website: www.marykay.com	

Merle Norman Cosmetics	color cosmetics
9130 Bellanca Avenue	skin care
Los Angeles, CA 90045	
phone: 310-641-3000	
fax: 310-641-7144	
website: www.merlenorman.com	

New Dana Perfumes Corporation	Chantilly
6353 W. Rogers Circle, Suite 1A	Cosmair
Boca Raton, FL 33487	Fetish
phone: 561-999-9918	Heaven Scent
fax: 561-999-8867	Love's Baby Soft
	Press and Go
	Tinkerbell

Princess Marcella Borghese	color cosmetics
180 Madison Avenue, Suite 506	fragrance
New York, NY 10016	skin care
phone: 212-659-5300 or 212-572-3100	
fax: 212-659-5301	
website: www.borghese.com	

Procter & Gamble
P.O. Box 599
Cincinnati, OH 45201
phone: 513-983-1100
fax: 513-983-8168
website: www.pg.com

Camay
Clearasil
Cover Girl
Giorgio Beverly Hills
Head & Shoulders
Hugo Boss
Laura Biagiotti-Roma
Max Factor
Noxzema
Oil of Olay
Pantene Pro-V
Pert Plus
Red
Secret
Sure
Vidal Sassoon

Revlon Consumer Products Corporation
625 Madison Avenue
New York, NY 10022
phone: 212-527-4000
fax: 212-527-4995
website: www.revlon.com

Almay
Charlie
Fire and Ice
Flex
Mitchum
Revlon
Ultima II

S. C. Johnson

1525 Howe Street

Racine, WI 53403

phone: 800-494-4855

fax: 262-260-4805

website: www.scjbrands.com

Skintimates

Shiseido Cosmetics (America) Ltd.

900 Third Avenue, Fifteenth Floor

New York, NY 10022

phone: 212-805-2300

fax: 212-688-0109

website: www.shiseido.com

color cosmetics

skin care

SkinMarket

3910 E. Royal Avenue, Unit B

Simi Valley, CA 93063

phone: 877-777-5576

fax: 805-527-3162

website: www.skinmarket.com

bath and body care

color cosmetics

hair care

nail care

Stephan Company

1850 W. McNab Road

Fort Lauderdale, FL 33309

phone: 954-971-0600

fax: 954-971-2633

website: www.thestephanco.com

Cashmere Bouquet

Frances Denney

Magic Wave

Stiff Stuff

Unilever

P.O. Box 68

Unilever House, Blackfriars

London, EC4P 4BQ

United Kingdom

phone: +44-20-7822-5252

fax: +44-20-7822-5951

website: www.unilever.com

House of Cerruti

House of Valentino

Pond's

Therma Silk

Vaseline

Urban Decay

729 Farad Street

Costa Mesa, CA 92627

phone: 949-631-4504

fax: 949-631-5986

website: www.urbandecay.com

color cosmetics

Victoria's Secret

P.O. Box 16589

Columbus, OH 43216

phone: 800-888-8200

fax: 614-337-5555

website: www.victoriassecret.com

bath and body care

fragrance

Yves Rocher, Inc.

P.O. Box 158

Champlain, NY 12919

phone: 888-909-0771

fax: 800-321-4909

website: www.yvesrocherusa.com

bath and body care

color cosmetics

fragrance

hair care

skin care

Appendix B: Resources

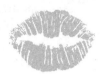

Bulk Herbs

Blessed Herbs
109 Barre Plains Road
Oakham, MA 01068
phone: 800-489-4372
fax: 508-882-3755
website: www.blessedherbs.com

Eureka Natural Foods
1626 Broadway
Eureka, CA 95501
phone: 800-603-8364
fax: 707-442-8199
website:
   www.eurekanaturalfoods.com

Glenbrook Farms
9228 169th Road
Live Oak, FL 32060
phone: 888-716-7627
fax: 904-362-6481
website:
   http://glenbrookfarm.com/herbs

Herb Corner
808 E. Strawbridge Avenue
Melbourne, FL 32901
phone: 321-768-1551
fax: 321-768-1567
website: www.herbcorner.net

Herb Shop
247 S.W. G Street
Grants Pass, OR 97526
phone: 541-479-3602
fax: 541-479-9550
website: www.bulkherbshop.com

Herbal and Traditional Healing
24 Ontario Street
Port Hope, ON, Canada L1A 2T6
phone: 905-885-3745
fax: 905-885-9837
website:
    www.herbalandtraditional.com

San Francisco Herb Company
250 Fourteenth Street
San Francisco, CA 94103
phone: 800-227-4530
fax: 415-861-4440
website: www.sfherb.com

Starwest Botanicals
11253 Trade Center Drive
Rancho Cordova, CA 95742
phone: 916-631-9755
fax: 916-853-9673
website:
    www.starwest-botanicals.com

Stony Mountain Botanicals
155 N. Water Street
Loudonville, OH 44842
phone: 888-994-4857
fax: 419-994-2128
website:
    www.wildroots.com/stony.htm

Essential Oils and Aromatherapy Equipment

Adriaflor
188 Lancaster Road
Walnut Creek, CA 94595
phone/fax: 925-933-3601
website:
    http://users.lanminds.com/ether

Altered States Herbs
200 N. Sixth Street
Reading, PA 19601
phone: 610-374-1552
fax: 610-374-2290
website:
    www.alteredstatesherbs.com

AromaLand
1326 Rufina Circle
Santa Fe, NM 84505
phone: 800-933-5267
fax: 505-438-7223
website:
    www.buyaromatherapy.com

Aroma-Pure
P.O. Box 1337
American Fork, UT 84003
phone: 888-826-2486
website: www.aroma-pure.com

Aromystique
P.O. Box 1482
Rockwall, TX 75087
phone: 888-722-1244
fax: 972-722-8082
website: www.aromystique.com

Aura Cacia
P.O. Box 311
Norway, IN 52318
phone: 800-437-3301
fax: 319-227-7966
website: www.auracacia.com

Australasian College of Herbal
  Studies
P.O. Box 57
Lake Oswego, OR 97034
phone: 800-487-8839
fax: 503-636-0706
website: www.herbed.com

Birch Hill Happenings
2898 County Road 103
Barnum, MN 55707
phone: 218-384-9294
fax: 218-384-3975
website:
  www.birchhillhappenings.com

Camden-Grey Essential Oils
7178-A S.W. Forty-Seventh Street
Miami, FL 33155
phone: 877-232-7662
fax: 305-740-8242
website: www.essentialoil.net

Dreaming Earth Botanicals
P.O. Box 727
Penrose, NC 28766
phone/fax: 800-897-8330
website: http://dreamingearth.com

Essential Oil Company
1719 S.E. Umatilla Street
Portland, OR 97202
phone: 800-729-5912
fax: 503-872-8767
website: http://essentialoil.com

Eureka Natural Foods
1626 Broadway
Eureka, CA 95501
phone: 800-603-8364
fax: 707-442-8199
website:
  www.eurekanaturalfoods.com

Indigo Wild
2131 Washington
Kansas City, MO 64108
phone: 800-361-5686
fax: 800-221-4035
website: www.indigowild.com

Jeanne Rose Aromatherapy
219 Carl Street
San Francisco, CA 94117
phone: 415-564-6785
fax: 415-564-6799
website: www.jeannerose.net

Mountain Rose Herbs
20818 High Street
North San Juan, CA 95960
phone: 800-879-3337
fax: 510-217-4012
website:
  www.mountainroseherbs.com

Natural Apothecary of Vermont
170 Whitney Hill Road
Brookline, VT 05345
phone: 802-365-7156
fax: 802-365-4029
website: www.organicoils.com

Rainbow Meadow
P.O. Box 457
Napoleon, MI 49261
phone: 800-207-4047
fax: 517-764-0940
website: www.rainbowmeadow.com

Spirit Scents
P.O. Box 941182
Plano, TX 75094
phone: 972-633-1679
website: www.spiritscents.com

Tisserand Aromatherapy
P.O. Box 750428
Petaluma, CA 94975
phone: 707-769-5120
fax: 707-769-0868
website: www.tisserand.com

Natural Cosmetics Companies

Abra Therapeutics
10365 Highway 116
Forestville, CA 94536
phone: 800-745-0761
fax: 707-869-9367
website: www.abratherapeutics.com

Annemarie Börlind
Börlind of Germany
P.O. Box 130
New London, NH 03257
phone: 800-447-7024
fax: 603-526-2074
website: www.borlind.com

Aubrey Organics
4419 N. Manhattan Avenue
Tampa, FL 33614
phone: 800-282-7394
fax: 813-876-8166
website: www.aubrey-organics.com

Aura Cacia
P.O. Box 311
Norway, IN 52318
phone: 800-437-3301
fax: 319-227-7966
website: www.auracacia.com

Auric Blends
P.O. Box 628
Graton, CA 95444
phone: 800-882-7247
fax: 707-829-3863
website: www.auricblends.com

Avalon Natural Products
1105 Industrial Avenue, #200
Petaluma, CA 94952
phone: 707-769-5120
fax: 707-769-0868
website:
   www.avalonnaturalproducts.com

Aztec Secret
P.O. Box 841
Parhump, NV 89041
phone: 775-727-8351
fax: 775-727-1882
website: www.aztec-secrets.com

Beeswork
122 Hamilton Drive, Suite D
Novato, CA 94949
phone: 415-883-5660
fax: 415-883-6038
website: www.beeswork.com

Better Botanicals
3066 M Street NW
Washington, DC 20007
phone: 888-224-3727
website: www.betterbotanicals.com

Bindi
P.O. Box 750-250
Forest Hills, NY 11375
phone: 800-952-4634
website: www.bindi.com

Botanics of California
P.O. Box 384
Ukiah, CA 95482
phone: 800-800-6141
fax: 707-462-0866
website:
   www.botanicscalifornia.com

Burt's Bees, Inc.
P.O. Box 13489
Durham, NC 27709
phone: 800-849-7112
fax: 800-429-7487
website: www.burtsbees.com

Color 'N Peel
P.O. Box 460
Harvard, NE 68944
phone: 402-463-3962
fax: 402-463-4476
website: www.colornpeel.com

Compliments of Nature
4717 Snowden Avenue
Lakewood, CA 90713
phone: 562-420-6127
fax: 526-420-6877
website: www.greenfeet.com

Deodorant Stones of America
9420 E. Doubletree Ranch Road,
   Unit 101
Scottsdale, AZ 85258
phone: 800-279-9318
fax: 480-451-5850
website: www.deodorantstones.com

Desert Essence
27460 Avenue Scott
Valencia, CA 91355
phone: 661-295-9601
fax: 661-232-5034
website: www.country-life.com

Dr. Hauschka Skin Care
  Preparations
59C North Street
Hatfield, MA 01038
phone: 800-247-9907
fax: 413-247-5633
website: www.drhauschka.com

Dreaming Earth Botanicals
P.O. Box 727
Penrose, NC 28766
phone: 800-897-8330
fax: 800-897-8330
website: www.dreamingearth.com

Dynamo House
P.O. Box 110
Richmond, 3121, Victoria
Australia
ACN 005 506 114
website: www.dynamoh.com.au

Earth Science
23705 Via Del Rio
Yorba Linda, CA 92687
phone: 800-222-6720
fax: 909-371-0509
website: www.earthscienceinc.com

Earthly Delights/Blue Cross Beauty
  Products
1251 Montague Street
Pacoima, CA 91331
phone: 818-896-8681
fax: 818-899-6420

Ecco Bella Botanicals
1133 Route 23
Wayne, NJ 07470
phone: 973-696-7766
fax: 973-696-7766
website:
  www.ecomall.com/biz/bella.htm

EO Small World Trading Company
15A Koch Road
Corte Madera, CA 94925
phone: 415-945-1900
fax: 415-945-1910
website: www.eoproducts.com

Essential Elements de la rue Verte
2675 Folsom Street
San Francisco, CA 94110
phone: 800-908-4009
fax: 415-920-0780
website: www.essentialelements.com

Faith in Nature Unit 5 Kay Street,
  Bury, Lancashire
BL9 6BU, United Kingdom
phone: +44 (0) 161-764-2555
fax: +44 (0) 161-762-9129
website:
  http://homepages.tesco.net/~faith
  products

Gabriel
P.O. Box 50130
Bellevue, WA 98015
phone: 800-497-6419
fax: 425-688-8665

Giovanni Hair Care and Cosmetics
21580 S. Wilmington Avenue
Long Beach, CA 90810
phone: 310-952-9960
fax: 310-952-9532
website:
  www.giovannicosmetics.com

Hemp Organics
P.O. Box 170507
San Francisco, CA 94117
phone: 415-861-4070
fax: 415-861-0943
website: www.colorganics.com

Home Health Products
P.O. Box 8425
Virginia Beach, VA 23450
phone: 800-284-9123
fax: 631-471-5693
website: www.puritan.com

Honeybee Gardens
311 South Street
Morgantown, PA 19543
phone: 888-478-9090
website:
  www.honeybeegardens.com

Igora Botanic
Hohenzollernring 127-129
D-22763 Hamburg, Germany
phone: 800-707-9997
fax: 040-8824-2312
website: www.schwarzkopf.de

Jakaré
P.O. Box 10124
Bozeman, MT 59719
phone: 877-525-2731
website: www.jakare.com

Jason Natural Cosmetics
8468 Warner Drive
Culver City, CA 90232
phone: 800-527-6605
fax: 310-838-9274
website: www.jason-natural.com

Kettle Care
6590 Farm to Market Road
Whitefish, MT 59937
phone: 406-862-9851
fax: 406-862-9851
website: www.kettlecare.com

Kiss My Face
P.O. Box 224
Gardiner, NY 12525
phone: 800-262-5477
fax: 845-255-4312
website: www.kissmyface.com

Light Mountain Henna/Lotus
  Brands
Box 325
Twin Lakes, WI 53181
phone: 800-824-6396
fax: 414-889-8591
website: www.internatural.com

Lily of Colorado
P.O. Box 12471
Denver, CO 80212
phone: 800-333-5459
website: www.lilyofcolorado.com

Logona USA, Inc.
554-E Riverside Drive
Asheville, NC 28801
phone: 828-252-9630
website: www.logona.com

Masada
P.O. Box 4767
North Hollywood, CA 91617
phone: 800-368-8811
fax: 818-717-8400
website: www.masada-spa.com

Mera
P.O. Box 218
Circle Pine, MN 55014
phone: 800-752-7261
fax: 763-767-1424

Moom
1574 Gulf Road, #1115A
Point Roberts, WA 98281
phone: 800-492-9464
fax: 604-241-0488
website: www.imoom.com

Mountain Rose Herbs
20818 High Street
North San Juan, CA 95960
phone: 800-879-3337
fax: 510-217-4012
website:
    www.mountainroseherbs.com

Nalz Water-Based Nail Polish
2143 Morris Avenue, #106
Union, NJ 07083
phone: 908-624-1989
website: www.nalz.com

Natural Beauty Watercolors Nail
    Polish
600 Twenty-Seventh Street South
St. Petersburg, FL 33712
phone: 888-664-5040
fax: 727-323-0456
website:
    www.naturalbeautycolors.com

Natural Crystal Deodorant
P.O. Box 14971
Austin, TX 78761
phone: 512-926-9662
fax: 512-926-1812
website: www.naturalcrystal.com

NaturElle Cosmetics Corporation
P.O. Box 9
Pine, CO 80470
phone: 800-442-3936
fax: 303-232-6880
website: www.naturalbeauty.com

Neways, Inc.
150 E. 400 N
Salem, UT 84653
phone: 801-423-2800
website: http://usa.neways.com

No-Miss Nail Care
6401 E. Rodgers Circle, Suite 14
Boca Raton, FL 33487
phone: 800-283-1963
fax: 561-994-6998
website: www.nomiss.com

Nonie of Beverly Hills
16158 Wyandotte Street
Van Nuys, CA 91406
phone: 888-666-4324
fax: 800-310-9004
website:
    www.nonieofbeverlyhills.com

Paul Penders
Blönbal Building, Temasya
    Industrial Park
Section U1, Jalan Glenmarie
40150 Shah Alam, Selangor,
    Malaysia
phone: 603-519-1888
fax: 603-519-1838
website: www.paulpenders.com.my

Penny Island
P.O. Box 521
Graton, CA 95444
phone: 707-823-2406
fax: 707-823-2506

Perfectly Beautiful
2419 N. Trenton
Mesa, AZ 85207
phone: 480-380-3053
fax: 480-380-2153
website:
    www.perfectlybeautiful.com

ProSeed/Imhotep, Inc.
P.O. Box 183
Ruby, NY 12475
phone: 800-677-8577
fax: 888-708-2686
website: www.imhotepinc.com

Rainbow Research
170 Wilbur Place
Bohemia, NY 11716
phone: 800-722-9595
fax: 631-589-4687
website: www.rainbowresearch.com

Real Purity
P.O. Box 307
Grass Lake, MI 49240
phone: 800-253-1694
fax: 517-522-3258
website: www.realpuritytm.com

Rich's
3721 S.E. 122nd Avenue
Portland, OR 97236
phone: 503-761-7450
fax: 503-761-5383
website: www.richdistributing.com

Simmons Natural Bodycare
42295 Highway 36
Bridgeville, CA 95526
phone: 707-777-1920
fax: 707-777-1920
website: http://home.pon.net/
   simmonsnaturals

Sue's Amazing/Sun Dog
P.O. Box 64
Westby, WI 54667
phone: 608-634-2988
fax: 608-634-2998

Terry and Company
300 W. Robles Avenue, #D
Santa Rosa, CA 95407
phone: 800-682-9224
fax: 707-538-3296
website: www.yakshifragrances.com

Touchme
3722 Bishop Strachan Court
Mississauga, ON, Canada L5N 6N9
phone: 905-785-7226
fax: 905-785-7232
website: www.touchme.ca

Trillium Herbal Company
185 E. Walnut Street
Sturgeon Bay, WI 54235
phone: 800-734-7253
fax: 920-746-7649
website: www.aromafusion.com

Urtekram
Klostermarken 20
DK-9550 Mraiager, Denmark
phone: +44 98-54-22-88
fax: +44 98-54-23-33
website: www.urtekram.com

VitaWave
2401 Eastman Avenue
Oxnard, CA 93003
phone: 805-981-1472
fax: 805-981-1492

V'tae Parfum & Body Care
571 Searls Avenue
Nevada City, CA 95959
phone: 800-643-3011
fax: 530-265-3709
website: www.vtae.com

Weleda
P.O. Box 249
Congers, NY 10920
phone: 800-289-1969
fax: 800-280-4899
website: www.weleda.com

Tools and Supplies

Burch Bottle and Packaging, Inc.
811 Tenth Street
Watervliet, NY 12189
phone: 800-903-2830
fax: 518-273-1846
website: www.burchbottle.com

Eureka Natural Foods
1626 Broadway
Eureka, CA 95501
phone: 800-603-8364
fax: 707-442-8199
website:
  www.eurekanaturalfoods.com

Lavender Lane
7337 #1 Roseville Road
Sacramento, CA 95842
phone: 888-593-4400
fax: 916-339-0842
website: www.lavenderlane.com

Mid Con
1465 N. Winchester
Olathe, KS 66061
phone: 800-547-1392
website: www.mid-conagri.com

Specialty Bottle Supply
2730 First Avenue South
Seattle, WA 98134
phone: 206-340-0459
fax: 206-903-0785
website: www.specialtybottle.com

Sunburst Bottle Company
5710 Auburn Boulevard, Suite 7
Sacramento, CA 95841
phone: 916-348-5576
fax: 916-348-3803
website: www.sunburstbottle.com

Suggested Reading

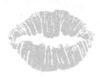

Berkson, D. Lindsey. *Hormone Deception.* Lincolnwood, Ill.: Contemporary
    Books, 2000.

Blumenthal, Mark, et al. *Herbal Medicine: Expanded Commission E Mono-*
    graphs. Newton, Mass.: Integrative Medicine Communications, 2000.

Colborn, Theo, et al. *Our Stolen Future: Are We Threatening Our Fertility,*
    Intelligence, and Survival? A Scientific Detective Story. New York:
    Plume, 1997.

Fagin, Dan, and Marianne Lavelle. *Toxic Deception: How the Chemical*
    Industry Manipulates Science, Bends the Law, and Endangers Your
    Health. Secaucus, N.J.: LPC, 1999.

Gibbs, Lois Marie. *Dying from Dioxin.* Boston: South End Press, 1995.

Gladstar, Rosemary. *Rosemary Gladstar's Herbs for Natural Beauty.* Pownal,
    Vt.: Storey Books, 1999.

Haas, Elson. *A Cookbook for All Seasons: A Healthy Eating Plan for Life.*
    Berkeley: Celestial Arts, 2000.

Keville, Kathi. *Herbs for Health and Healing.* Emmaus, Pa.: Rodale Press,
    1996.

Krimsky, Sheldon, and Lynn Goldman. *Hormonal Chaos: The Scientific and*
    Social Origins of Environmental Endocrine Hypothesis. Baltimore:
    Johns Hopkins University Press, 1999.

Lawless, Julia. *The Illustrated Encyclopedia of Essential Oils: The Complete Guide to the Use of Oils in Aromatherapy and Herbalism.* London: Thorsons Publishing, 1995.

Rose, Jeanne. *Jeanne Rose: Herbal Body Book: The Herbal Way to Natural Beauty and Health for Men and Women.* Berkeley: Frog, 2000.

Schettler, Ted, et al. *Generations at Risk: Reproductive Health and the Environment.* Cambridge: MIT Press, 1999.

Stauber, John, and Sheldon Rampton. *Toxic Sludge Is Good for You! Lies, Damn Lies, and the Public Relations Industry.* Monroe, Mass.: Common Courage Press, 1995.

Wildwood, Christine. *Encyclopedia of Aromatherapy.* Rochester, Vt.: Inner Traditions International, 1996.

Winter, Ruth. *A Consumer's Dictionary of Cosmetic Ingredients.* New York: Three Rivers Press, 1999.

Literary Credits

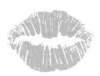

Pages v and 14: Excerpts from *Silent Spring* by Rachel Carson. Copyright © 1962 by Rachel L. Carson, renewed 1990 by Roger Christie. Reprinted by permission of Houghton Mifflin Co. All rights reserved.

Page xvi: Paula Begoun, *The Beauty Bible* (Seattle: Beginning Press, 1997).

Page 6: John Stauber and Sheldon Rampton, *Toxic Sludge Is Good for You* (Monroe, Maine: Common Courage Press, 1995).

Page 15: Blanche Wiesen Cook, *Eleanor Roosevelt*, vol. 2, *The Defining Years* (New York: Penguin Putnam, Inc., 1999).

Page 16: Sheila Kaplan, "The Ugly Face of the Cosmetics Lobby," *Ms.*, January/February 1994, 88–9. Reprinted by permission of *Ms.* magazine, ©1994.

Page 16: Ruth Winter, *A Consumer's Dictionary of Cosmetic Ingredients* (New York: Three Rivers Press, 1999).

Page 82: Samuel S. Epstein, M.D., "Major Cosmetic and Toiletry Ingredient Poses Avoidable Cancer Risks," Cancer Prevention Coalition (22 February 1998).

Page 162: James Duke, Ph.D., *The Green Pharmacy* (Emmaus, Pa.: Rodale Press, 1997).

Notes

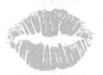

Chapter 1

1. H. Mielke et al., "Lead-Based Hair Products: Too Hazardous for House-hold Use," *Journal of American Pharmaceutical Association* NS37 (January/February 1997): 85–9.
2. R. Winter, *A Consumer's Dictionary of Cosmetic Ingredients* (New York: Three Rivers Press, 1999).
3. Winter.
4. R. Freedman, *Beauty Bound* (New York: Lexington Books, 1986).
5. Winter.
6. Winter.
7. "Preliminary Results for the Fifty-Three Weeks to 3 March 2001," The Body Shop International PLC, 2 May 2001.
8. "Community Trade: What You Buy Can Make a Difference," The Body Shop.
9. J. Stauber and S. Rampton, *Toxic Sludge Is Good for You* (Monroe, Maine: Common Courage Press, 1995).
10. J. Entine, "The Queen of Bubble Bath," *Brazzil*, December 1996, 19.
11. Entine.
12. "Preliminary Results."
13. "What's Wrong with The Body Shop?" London Greenpeace, 21 March 1998.

14. "Aveda: Creating a Healthy Business," *Drug and Cosmetic Industry* 161 (1 August 1997): 16–9.
15. "Aveda: Creating a Healthy Business."
16. D. Hendy, "The Green Theory: Facing the Challenge of Environmentally Friendly Packaging in the 'Natural Products' Market," *Drug and Cosmetic Industry* 158 (February 1996): 26–9.
17. "Aveda: The Scoop," Vault. Available at www.vault.com.
18. S. Kaplan, "The Ugly Face of the Cosmetics Lobby," *Ms.*, January/February 1994, 88–9.
19. S. Dentel et al., "Effects of Surfactants on Sludge Dewatering and Pollutant Fate," Department of Civil Engineering, University of Delaware, 1 August 1993.
20. "Alkylphenolic Compounds," Friends of the Earth, Scotland, 17 December 1998.
21. "Reproductive Tract Abnormalities," *Reproductive Effects*, World Wildlife Fund. Available at www.wwfcanada.org.
22. "Immune Function Effects," World Wildlife Fund. Available at www.wwfcanada.org.
23. T. Colborn et al., *Our Stolen Future* (New York: Plume, 1997).
24. P. Frazer, "Why Your Recycling Helps," *News on Earth*, June 1999.
25. People for the Ethical Treatment of Animals. Available at www.peta.org.
26. "The Draize Test: Blinding for Beauty," People for the Ethical Treatment of Animals, Fact Sheet No. 10.
27. "The Draize Eye Irritancy Test," Doris Day Animal League.
28. "LD50 Test: Lethal Limits," People for the Ethical Treatment of Animals, Fact Sheet No. 9.
29. "Facts on the Draize Eye and Skin Irritancy Tests," National Antivivisection Society.
30. *Beyond the Draize Test* (Washington, D.C.: Physicians Committee for Responsible Medicine).
31. *Cosmetic Testing*, People for the Ethical Treatment of Animals.
32. "Product Safety Testing at Procter & Gamble," P&G Public Affairs Division, 1995.
33. "What Procter & Gamble Doesn't Want You to Know About This Toothpaste," In Defense of Animals.
34. "Companies That Test on Animals," People for the Ethical Treatment of Animals. Available at www.peta-online.org.

35. "Draize Test Is Done to Limit Liability," Beyond the Draize Test (Washington, D.C.: Physicians Committee for Responsible Medicine), 6.

Chapter 2

1. R. Carson, *Silent Spring* (New York: Houghton Mifflin, 1962).
2. I. Franck and D. Brownstone, *The Green Encylopedia* (New York: Prentice Hall, 1992).
3. S. Kaplan, "The Ugly Face of the Cosmetics Lobby," *Ms.*, January/February 1994, 88–9.
4. "FDA Authority over Cosmetics," U.S. Food and Drug Administration Center for Food Safety and Applied Nutrition, Office of Cosmetics and Colors, 3 February 1995.
5. J. Levitt, "Restoration of Voluntary Cosmetic Registration Program," U.S. Food and Drug Administration Center for Food Safety and Applied Nutrition, 23 December 1998.
6. B. Cook, *Eleanor Roosevelt*, vol. 2, *The Defining Years* (New York: Penguin Putnam, Inc., 1999).
7. R. Winter, *A Consumer's Dictionary of Cosmetic Ingredients* (New York: Three Rivers Press, 1999).
8. "FDA Authority over Cosmetics."
9. C. Lewis, "Prohibited Ingredients," *FDA Consumer*, May/June 1998.
10. Kaplan.
11. "Toxicity Testing: Strategies to Determine Needs and Priorities," National Research Council, Washington, D.C., National Academy Press, 1984.
12. R. Garrison and E. Somer, *The Nutrition Desk Reference* (New Canaan, CT: Keats Publishing, 1995).
13. P. Balch and J. Balch, *Prescription for Nutritional Healing* (New York: Avery, 2000).
14. "Look Good . . . Feel Better," Cosmetic, Toiletry, and Fragrance Association. Available at www.lookgoodfeelbetter.org/1.00.html.
15. G. Rimkus and M. Wolf, "Polycyclic Musk Fragrances in Human Adipose Tissue and Human Milk," *Chemosphere* 33, no. 10 (1996): 2033–43.
16. L. Gibbs, *Dying from Dioxin* (Boston: South End Press, 1995).
17. T. Hawkins, "Dioxin Fact Sheet," National Institute of Environmental Health Sciences, Washington, D.C., September 1994.

18. T. Colborn et al., *Our Stolen Future* (New York: Plume, 1997).
19. "Alkylphenolic Compounds," Friends of the Earth. Available at http://website.lineone.net/~mwarhurst/apeintro.html.
20. E. Routledge et al., "Some Alkyl Hydroxy Benzoate Preservatives (Parabens) Are Estrogenic," *Toxicology and Applied Pharmacology* 153 (1998): 12–19.
21. K. Pedersen et al., "The Preservatives Ethyl-, Propyl-, and Butylparaben Are Oestrogenic in an In Vivo Fish Assay," *Pharmacological Toxicology* 86 (2000 March): 110–13.
22. "Toxic Toy Story," Greenpeace U.S.A. Available at www.greenpeace usa.org.
23. D. Stehlin, "Cosmetic Safety: More Complex than at First Blush," *FDA Consumer*, November 1991.
24. "Organic Cosmetics," Environmental News Network, "ENN Daily News," 1 August 1996.
25. Stehlin.
26. Winter.
27. D. Steinman and S. Epstein, *The Safe Shopper's Bible* (New York: Macmillan, 1995).
28. Senate, Kennedy, FDA Reform and Cosmetic Preemption, 5 September 1997.
29. Winter.
30. Winter.
31. Winter.
32. Winter.
33. Winter.
34. Winter.
35. Winter.
36. Winter.
37. Winter.
38. D. Fagin and M. Lavelle, *Toxic Deception* (Secaucus, N.J.: LPC, 1999).
39. Winter.
40. A. Hampton, *What's in Your Cosmetics?* (Tucson: Odonian Press, 1995).
41. Balch and Balch.
42. H. Mielke et al., "Lead-Based Hair Products: Too Hazardous for Household Use," *Journal of American Pharmaceutical Association* NS37 (January/February 1997): 85–9.
43. T. Schettler et al., *Generations at Risk* (Cambridge: MIT Press, 1999).

44. "Group Sues Hair Dye Maker, Demands Lead," Reuters, 1 February 1997.
45. Hampton.
46. Winter.
47. *The Medical Post*, 27 September 1994.
48. *Human Reproduction*, February 1990.
49. Material Safety Data Sheet: Propylene Glycol. Available at www.http://chem-course.ucsd.edu/cou./propyleneglycol.-fisher.htm.
50. Winter.
51. Winter.
52. "Dangerous Beauty," *New Health and Longevity*, February 1994.
53. "Dangerous Beauty."
54. *Drug and Cosmetic Industry*, November 1992.
55. "Cook Study Suggests Link Between Ovarian Cancer, Genital Powders, Sprays," Fred Hutchinson Cancer Research Center Newsletter, 3 April 1997.
56. Winter.
57. Schettler et al.
58. Winter.
59. "Synthetic Vitamin E Cannot Bear 'Natural' Labeling," *Nutrition Science News*, June 1996: 6.

Chapter 3

1. R. Winter, *A Consumer's Dictionary of Cosmetic Ingredients* (New York: Three Rivers Press, 1999).

Chapter 4

1. R. Winter, *A Consumer's Dictionary of Cosmetic Ingredients* (New York: Three Rivers Press, 1999).
2. Winter.
3. "Alpha Hydroxy Acids in Cosmetics," U.S. Food and Drug Administration, 3 July 1997.
4. K. Erickson, "ACE Your Face," *GreatLife*, January 2000, 48–50.
5. K. Keller and N. Fenske, "Uses of Vitamins A, C, and E and Related Compounds in Dermatology: A Review," *Journal of the American Academy of Dermatology* 1998: 611–25.

6. S. Lamm, M.D., clinical assistant professor of medicine, New York University, School of Medicine. Telephone interview with author, 3 November 1997.

7. M. Bykowski, "Zinc Oxide Offers Broad Protection Against UVA," *Skin and Allergy News* 28 (1997): 26.

8. D. Stoll, M.D., fellow of the American Academy of Dermatology. Telephone interview with author, 14 December 1997.

9. C. Wu, "Melanoma Madness," *Science News* 153, no. 23 (1998): 360. J. Knowland et al., "Sunlight-Induced Mutagenicity of a Common Sunscreen Ingredient," *FEBS Letters* 324 (1993): 309–13. P. McHugh, "Characterization of DNA Damage Inflicted by Free Radicals from a Mutagenic Sunscreen Ingredient and Its Location Using an In Vitro Genetic Reversion Assay," *Photochemistry and Photobiology* 66 (1997): 276–81.

10. "Sunscreen Absorption," *Skin and Allergy News* 28 (1997): 62.

11. C. Garland and F. Garland, "Effects of Sunscreens on UV Radiation-Induced Enhancement of Melanoma Growth in Mice," *Journal of the National Cancer Institute* 86 (1994): 798–801.

12. P. Autier et al., "Quantity of Sunscreen Used by European Students," *British Journal of Dermatology* 144 (2001): 288–91.

13. T. Donegan, CTFA letter to FDA regarding final regulation for sunscreen drug products, 24 May 2000.

14. "Sunscreens May Not Protect Against Melanoma Skin Cancer," Memorial Sloan-Kettering Cancer Center Press Release, 17 February 1998.

15. G. Ainsleigh, "Beneficial Effects of Sun Exposure on Cancer Mortality," *Preventative Medicine* 22 (1993): 132–40.

16. A. Raman et al., "Antimicrobial Effects of Tea Tree Oil and Its Major Components on *Staphylococcus aureus, Staph. epidermidis,* and Propionibacterium Acnes," *Letters in Applied Microbiology* 21 (1995): 242–5.

17. Winter.

18. Winter.

Chapter 5

1. D. Steinman and S. Epstein, *The Safe Shopper's Bible* (New York: Macmillan, 1995).

2. R. Winter, *A Consumer's Dictionary of Cosmetic Ingredients* (New York: Three Rivers Press, 1999).

3. M. Prinsen et al., "Skin Sensitization Testing: The Relevance of Rechallenge and Pretreatment with Sodium Lauryl Sulfate in the Guinea Pig Maximization Test," *Food and Chemical Toxicology* 37 (1997): 267.

4. S. Epstein, M.D., "Major Cosmetic and Toiletry Ingredient Poses Avoidable Cancer Risks," Cancer Prevention Coalition, 22 February 1998.

5. Epstein.

6. "Diethanolamine and Cosmetic Products," U.S. Food and Drug Administration Center for Food Safety and Applied Nutrition, Office of Cosmetics Fact Sheet, 9 December 1999.

7. "Toxicology and Carcinogenesis Studies of Lauric Acid Diethanolamine Condensate in F344/N Rats and B6C3F$_1$ Mice (Dermal Studies)," National Toxicology Program, NIEHS, NIH, 9 December 1997. "Final Study Report: Developmental Toxicity Screen for Diethanolamine (CAS No. 111-42-2). Administered by Gavage to Sprague-Dawley (CD) Rats on Gestational Days 6 Through 19: Evaluation of Dams and Pups Through Postnatal Day 21," National Toxicology Program, NIEHS, NIH, 22 December 1999.

8. Senate, Kennedy, FDA Reform and Cosmetic Preemption, 5 September 1997.

9. Winter.

10. M. Thun et al., "Hair Dye Use and Risk of Fatal Cancer in U.S. Women," *Journal of the National Cancer Institute* 86 (1994): 210–5.

11. D. Sandler et al., "Hair Dye Use and Leukemia." *American Journal of Epidemiology* 138 (1993): 363–7.

12. A. Tzonou et al., "Hair Dyes, Analgesics, Tranquilizers, and Perineal Talc Application as Risk Factors for Ovarian Cancer," *International Journal of Cancer* 55 (1993): 408–10.

13. Winter.

14. L. Cook et al., "Hair Product Use and the Risk of Breast Cancer in Young Women," *Cancer Causes Control* 10 (1999): 551–9.

15. Senate, Kennedy.

16. A. Belton and T. Chira, "Fatal Anaphylactic Reaction to Hair Dye," *American Journal of Forensic Medicine and Pathology* 18 (1997): 290–92.

17. Winter.

18. S. Prahalada et al., "Effects of Finasteride, a Type 2 5-Alpha Reductase Inhibitor, on Fetal Development in the Rhesus Monkey (*Macaca mulatta*)," *Teratology* 55 (1997): 119–31.

19. G. Pogatsa-Murray et al., "Changes in Left Ventricular Mass During Treatment with Minoxidil and Cilazapril in Hypertensive Patients with Left Ventricular Hypertrophy," *Journal of Human Hypertension* 11 (1997): 149–56.

Chapter 6

1. "How Fit Are Your Feet?" American Podiatric Medical Association. Available at www.apma.org/75m.htm.
2. J. McConnaughey, "Half of All Soaps Are Antibacterial," Associated Press, 11 September 2000.
3. T. Schettler et al., *Generations at Risk* (Cambridge: MIT Press, 1999).
4. M. Schorr, "Clean Freaks?" ABCNews.com, 7 September 2000. Available at http://abcnews.go.com/sections/living/dailynews/soaps000907.html.
5. L. McMurry et al., "Triclosan Targets Lipid Synthesis," *Nature* 394 (1998): 831–2.
6. P. Costner, senior scientist, Greenpeace. Telephone interview with author, 17 April 2001.
7. Schettler et al.
8. A. Schecter et al., "2,3,7,8 Chlorine Substituted Dioxin and Dibenzofuran Congeners in 2,4-D, 2,4,5-T, and Pentachlorophenol," *Organohalogen Cpds* 32 (1997): 51–5.
9. "Undisclosed Carcinogens in Cosmetics and Personal Care Products Pose Avoidable Risks of Cancer, Warns Samuel Epstein, M.D.," PR Newswire, 16 January 2001.
10. "Lanolin Contaminated with Pesticides," U.S. Food and Drug Administration, 13 September 1988. Available at http://fa.gov/bbs/topics/answers/ans00215.html.
11. R. Winter, *A Consumer's Dictionary of Cosmetic Ingredients* (New York: Three Rivers Press, 1999).
12. T. Batten et al., "Contact Dermatitis from the Old Formula E45 Cream," *Contact Dermatitis* 30 (1994): 159–61.
13. B. Vazquez et al., "Antiinflammatory Activity of Extracts from Aloe Vera Gel," *Journal of Ethnopharmacology* 55 (1996): 69–75.
14. P. Balch and J. Balch, *Prescription for Nutritional Healing* (New York: Avery, 2000).
15. Balch and Balch.
16. "Toluene," Agency for Toxic Substances and Disease Registry, 1995.

17. "Chemicals in the Environment: Toluene (CAS No. 108-88-3)," U.S. Environmental Protection Agency Office of Pollution Prevention and Toxics, 1994.
18. T. Gotohda et al., "Effect of Toluene Inhalation on Astrocytes and Neurotrophic Factor in Rat Brain," *Forensic Science International* 113 (2000): 233–8.
19. T. Ng et al., "Risk of Spontaneous Abortion in Workers Exposed to Toluene," *British Journal of Industrial Medicine* 49 (1992): 804–8.
20. Winter.
21. "An Update on Formaldehyde: 1997 Revision," Consumer Product Safety Commission, CPSC Document No. 725. Available at www.cpsc.gov/cpscpub/pubs/725.html.
22. Winter.
23. I. Colon et al., "Identification of Phthalate Esters in the Serum of Young Puerto Rican Girls with Premature Breast Development," *Environmental Health Perspectives* 108 (2000): 895–900.
24. B. Blout et al., "Levels of Seven Urinary Phtalate Metabolites in a Human Reference Population," *Environmental Health Perspectives* 108 (2000): 972–82.
25. Winter.
26. Industry statistics, *Nail* magazine.
27. A. Spencer et al., "Control of Ethyl Methacrylate Exposures During the Application of Artificial Fingernails," *American Industrial Hygiene Association Journal* 58 (1997): 214–8.
28. "Methyl Ethyl Ketone," Material Safety Data Sheet, Strategic Services Division, Mallinckrodt Baker, Inc., 15 September 1998.
29. "Methy Ethyl Ketone," Hazardous Substance Fact Sheet, New Jersey Department of Health and Senior Services Right to Know Program, Trenton, N.J.
30. S. Hedderwick et al., "Pathogenic Organisms Associated with Artificial Fingernails Worn by Health Care Workers," *Infection Control and Hospital Epidemiology* 21 (2000): 505–9.
31. D. Blumenthal, "Artificial Nail Remover Poses Poisoning Risk," *FDA Consumer*, June 1989.
32. D. Steinman and S. Epstein, *The Safe Shopper's Bible* (New York: Macmillan, 1995).

33. "Update on Artificial Nail Removers," U.S. Food and Drug Administration Center for Food Safety and Applied Nutrition, Office of Cosmetics and Colors, December 1999.
34. "Acetonitrile," Hazardous Substance Fact Sheet, New Jersey Department of Health and Senior Services Right to Know Program, Trenton, N.J.
35. Z. Draelos, meeting of the American Academy of Dermatology, 1997.
36. J. Guin et al., "Contact Sensitization to Cyanoacrylate Adhesive as a Cause of Severe Onychodystrophy," *International Journal of Dermatology* 37 (1998): 31–6.
37. P. Balch and J. Balch, *Prescription for Nutritional Healing* (New York: Avery, 2000).
38. C. Jansen et al., "Effects of Fingernail Length and Hand Performance," *Journal of Hand Therapy* 13 (2000): 211–7.
39. "Foot Faqs," American Podiatric Medical Association. Available at www.apma.org/faq.html.
40. B. Rowlands, "Well-Being: Put Your Best Foot Forward," *Daily Telegraph*, 28 May 1999, 24.
41. Winter.
42. Winter.
43. "Beauty Salon Health Risks?" Health Education Program, Columbia University, 23 May 1997. Available at www. goaskalice.columbia .edu/1191.html.

Chapter 7

1. P. Begoun, *The Beauty Bible* (Seattle: Beginning Press, 1997).
2. R. Winter, *A Consumer's Dictionary of Cosmetic Ingredients* (New York: Three Rivers Press, 1999).
3. R. Wester et al., "In Vivo Percutaneous Absorption of Boronas Boric Acid, Borax, and Disodium Octaborate Tetrahydrate in Humans: A Summary," *Biological Trace Element Research* 66 (1998): 101–9.
4. Winter.
5. Winter.
6. B. Sansal, "The Turkish Bath," Available at www.geocities.com/the tropics/paradise/5831/hamam.htm.
7. E. Sainio et al., "Ingredients and Safety of Cellulite Creams," *European Journal of Dermatology* 10 (2000): 596–603.
8. Winter.

9. L. Bryld et al., "Iodopropynyl Butylcarbamate: A New Contact Allergen," *Contact Dermatitis* 36 (1997): 156–8.

10. Winter.

11. Begoun.

12. D. Goldberg, "Hair Removal Techniques Options," Health Focus Interview transcript, 14 August 2000. Available at http://my.webmd.com/content/article/1700.50986.

13. Information Resources, Inc., Chicago, 1996.

14. J. Duke, Ph.D., *The Green Pharmacy* (Emmaus, PA: Rodale Press, 1997).

15. E. Haas, M.D., founder and director, The Preventive Medical Center of Marin. Telephone interviews with author, January–April 1998.

16. Winter.

17. T. Kruck, Ph.D., associate professor of physiology (ret.), University of Toronto, Canada. Telephone interview with author, 7 April 1998.

18. W. Pendlebury, M.D., professor of pathology, College of Medicine, University of Vermont. Telephone interview with author, 9 April 1998.

19. "Aerosol Propellant Gas Shown Toxic to Animals," *Lab Animal* 2 (September/October 1998): 5.

20. L. Cook et al., "Perineal Powder Exposure and the Risk of Ovarian Cancer," *American Journal of Epidemiology* 145 (1997): 459–65.

21. "Yeast Vaginitis," University Health Center, University of Maryland, College Park.

Chapter 8

1. C. Nasel et al., "Functional Imaging of Effects of Fragrances on the Human Brain After Prolonged Inhalation," *Chemical Senses* 19 (1994): 359–64.

2. V. MacDonald, "The Fine Fragrance Market," *Household and Personal Products on the Internet*, April 2000.

3. M. Mogelonsky, "Dollars and Scents," *American Demographics*, June 1997.

4. C. Canning, "Fine Fragrance," *Household and Personal Products on the Internet*, November 1996.

5. Committee on Science and Technology, U.S. House of Representatives, Report 99-827, 16 September 1986.

6. "The Sweet Smell of Success," *The Economist*, 5 September 1998, 75.

7. L. Wallace et al., "Identification of Polar Volatile Organic Compounds in Consumer Products and Common Microenvironments," Environmental Protection Agency, Paper No. A312, 1 March 1991.
8. Aldrich MSDS Database. Available at www.sigma-aldrich.com.
9. Aldrich MSDS Database.
10. Aldrich MSDS Database.
11. J. Lessenger, "Occupational Acute Anaphylactic Reaction to Assault by Perfume Spray in the Face," *Journal of the American Board of Family Practice* 14 (2001): 137–40.
12. Gibson et al., "Social Support in Persons with Self-Reported Sensitivity to Chemicals," *Research in Nursing and Health* 21 (1998): 103–15.
13. R. Anderson and J. Anderson, "Acute Toxic Effects of Fragrance Products," *Archives of Environmental Health* 53 (1998): 138–46.
14. T. Lorig, "EEG and ERP Studies of Low-Level Odor Exposure in Normal Subjects," *Toxicology and Industrial Health* 10 (1994): 579–86.
15. "Facts About Asthma," ARC Report 2000, American Lung Association. Available at www.lungusa.org.
16. E. Millqvist and O. Lowhagen, "Placebo-Controlled Challenges with Perfume in Patients with Asthmalike Symptoms," *Allergy* 51 (1996): 434–9.
17. P. Kumar et al., "Inhalation Challenge Effects of Perfume Scent Strips in Patients with Asthma," *Annals of Allergy, Asthma, and Immunology* 75 (1995): 429–33.
18. S. Lehrer, "Asthmatics' Reactions to Common Perfumes," American Academy of Allergy, Asthma, and Immunology Annual Meeting, 3–8 March 2000.
19. "Allergies: Culprit Could Be in Cosmetic Bag," American Academy of Dermatology, 11 March 2000.
20. Migraine Relief Center, Glaxo-Wellcome. Available at www.migrainehelp.com.
21. M. Coseman and T. Burchfield, "Migraines: Myth Versus Reality," Migraine Awareness Group: A National Understanding for Migraineurs. Available at www.migraines.org.
22. Nasel et al.
23. Lorig.
24. P. Scheinman, "Is It Really Fragrance-Free?" *American Journal of Contact Dermatitis* 8 (1997): 239–42.

25. "Fragrance-Free and Unscented," U.S. Food and Drug Administration Center for Food Safety and Applied Nutrition, Office of Cosmetics and Colors, 19 December 1994.
26. M. Gomes-Carneiro et al., "Mutagenicity Testing (+/−) -Camphor, 1,8-Cineole, Citral, Citronellal, (−)-Menthol, and Terpineol with the Salmonella/Microsome Assay," *Mutation Research* 416 (1998): 129–36.
27. R. Bronaugh et al., "Dermal Exposure Assessment for the Fragrance Musk Xylol," Abstract No. 274, *Proceedings of the Society of Toxicology*, 1998 Annual Meeting.
28. F. Rimkus and M. Wolf, "Polycyclic Musk Fragrance in Human Adipose Tissue and Human Milk," *Chemosphere* 33 (1996): 2033–43. B. Liebl and S. Ehrenstorfer, "Nitro-Musk Compounds in Breast Milk," *Gesundheitswesen* 55 (1993): 527–32.
29. J. Riedel et al., "Haemoglobin Binding of a Musk Xylene Metabolite in Man," *Xenobiotica* 29 (1999): 573–82.
30. "Glycol Esters," HESIS Fact Sheet No. 8, Hazard Evaluation System and Information Service, Berkeley, January 1989.
31. T. Schettler et al., *Generations at Risk* (Cambridge: MIT Press, 1999). "Tert-Butanol," MSDS, CAS No. 75-65-0, Aldrich.
32. T. Yamagishi et al., "Identification of Musk Xylene and Musk Ketone in Freshwater Fish Collected from the Tama River, Tokyo," *Bulletin of Environmental Contamination and Toxicology* 26 (1981): 565–662.
33. C. Daughton and T. Ternes, "Pharmaceuticals and Personal Care Products in the Environment: Agents of Subtle Change?" *Environmental Health Perspectives* 107, Sup. 6 (December 1999).
34. C. Rimkus, "Polycyclic Musk Fragrances in the Aquatic Environment," *Toxicology Letter* 111 (1999): 37–56.
35. D. Herren and J. Berset, "Nitro Musks, Nitro Musk Amino Metabolites, and Polycyclic Musks in Sewage Sludges: Quantitative Determination by HRGC-Ion-Trap-MS/MS and Mass Spectral Characterization of the Amino Metabolites," *Chemosphere* 40 (2000): 565–74. J. Berset et al., "Analysis of Nitro Musk Compounds and Their Amino Metabolites in Liquid Sewage Sludges Using NMR and Mass Spectrometry," *Analytical Chemistry* 72 (2000): 2124–31.
36. Daughton and Ternes.
37. J. Manura, "The Analysis of Perfumes and Their Effect on Indoor Air Pollution," Scientific Instrument Services, November 1989.

38. R. Kallenborn et al., "Gas Chromatographic Determination of Synthetic Musk Compounds in Norwegian Air Samples," *Journal of Chromatography* A 846 (1999): 295–306.

39. H. Wisneski Havery and C. Donald, "Nitro Musks in Fragrance Products: An Update of Findings," *Cosmetics and Toiletries* 111, no. 6 (June 1996): 73–6. "FDA Authority over Cosmetics," U.S. Food and Drug Administration Center for Food Safety and Applied Nutrition, Office of Cosmetics and Colors, 3 February 1995.

40. B. Bridges, "Self-Regulation of the Fragrance Industry Is Inadequate at Best," *Flipside Alternative Daily* 2 (October 1999).

41. P. Frosh, J. Johansen, and I. White, eds., *Fragrances: Beneficial and Adverse Effects* (New York: Springer Verlag, 1998).

42. B. Bridges, "Industry Self-Regulation." Available at www.ameliaww .com/fpin/indselreg.htm.

43. C. Guttman, "Contact Allergies: Voluntary Labeling of Fragrance Allergens Needed," *Dermatology Times* 20 (1 August 1999): 33.

44. P. Spencer et al., "Fragrance Exposure Causes Aggression Hyperactivity and Nerve Damage," *Neurotoxicology* 1 (1979): 221–37.

45. P. Spencer et al., "Common Fragrance Ingredient Damages Connections Between Brain Cells," *Toxicology and Applied Pharmacology* 75 (1984): 571–5.

46. "Prohibited Ingredients and Related Safety Issues," U.S. Food and Drug Administration Center for Food Safety and Applied Nutrition, Office of Cosmetics and Colors, 30 March 2000.

47. W. Schriber et al., "Flavors and Fragrances: The Chemistry Challenges," *Chemtech* 27 (1997): 58–62.

48. "Hundreds of Consumers Ask FDA to Put Warning Labels on Eternity Perfume: EHN Finds Hazardous Chemicals in Designer Fragrance," Environmental Health Network Press Release, 18 August 1999.

49. S. Epstein, M.D., "Perfume: Cupid's Arrow or Poison Dart," Cancer Prevention Coalition/Environmental Health Network Joint Press Release, 7 February 2000.

50. "Excessive Use of Fragrance Products in Public Places," Sierra Club, San Francisco Chapter, Conservation Committee Resolution 98.12.01 (December 1998). D. Franz and H. Prall, "Smelling Good But Feeling Bad," *E Magazine*, January/February 2000.

51. "Access Board Adopts Fragance-Free Policy; Strong Recommendations for Future Action on MCS for FY 2001," National Center for Environmental Health Strategies, 26 July 2000.

52. "Dancing in Clean Air: Our Fragrance-Free Policy," Seattle Folklore Society. Available at www.scar.rad.washington.edu/ball99/fragrance .html.

53. Franz and Prall.

54. D. Ryman, *Aromatherapy: The Complete Guide to Plant and Flower Essences for Health and Beauty* (New York: Bantam Books, 1993).

55. V. Horn, "Bathed in Fragrance." *GreatLife*, January 1999, 50–2.

56. R. Winter, *A Consumer's Dictionary of Cosmetic Ingredients* (New York: Three Rivers Press, 1999).

57. "What Is CO_2 Extraction?" Nature's Gift Aromatherapy Products. Available at www.naturesgift.com/co2.htm.

58. S. Pearce, "What Are Essential Oils and How Do They Work?" Britannia Natural Products Ltd. Available at www.cotpubco.demon.co.uk/cosweb/ wheyssoil.html.

59. M. Lis-Balchin, "Essential Oils and 'Aromatherapy': Their Modern Role in Healing." *Journal of the Royal Society of Health* 117 (1997): 324–9.

60. M. Diego et al., "Aromatherapy Positively Affects Mood, EEG Patterns of Alertness, and Math Computations," *International Journal of Neuroscience* 96 (1998): 217–24. Saeki, "The Effect of Footbath with or Without the Essential Oil of Lavender on the Autonomic Nervous System: A Randomized Trial," *Complementary Therapies in Medicine* 8 (2000): 2–7.

61. J. Buckle, "Use of Aromatherapy as a Complementary Treatment for Chronic Pain," *Alternative Therapies in Health and Medicine* 5 (1999): 42–51. D. Walsh, "Using Aromatherapy in the Management of Psoriasis," *Nursing Standards* 11 (1996): 53–6. I. Hay et al., "Randomized Trial of Aromatherapy: Successful Treatment for Alopecia Areata," *Archives of Dermatology* 134 (1998): 1349–52.

Chapter 9

1. "So what about THIS lipstick?" Coty, *Harper's Bazaar*, 1935.

2. A. Verrill, *Perfumes and Spices: Including an Account of Soaps and Cosmetics* (New York: L. C. Page and Co., 1940).

3. J. Henkel, "From Shampoo to Cereal: Seeing to the Safety of Color Additives," *FDA Consumer*, December 1993.

4. "Report on the Certification of Color Additives, Foreign and Domestic Manufacturers: FY 2001—First Quarter." U.S. Food and Drug Administration Center for Food Safety and Applied Nutrition, Office of Cosmetics and Colors. Available at http://vm.cfsan.fda.gov.

5. R. Winter, *A Consumer's Dictionary of Cosmetic Ingredients* (New York: Three Rivers Press, 1999).

6. "Appendix A: Color Additive Status List," Office of Regulatory Affairs, Inspectional References, Investigations Operations Manual, U.S. Food and Drug Administration, 2001.

7. Winter.

8. D. Blumenthal, "Red No. 3 and Other Colorful Controversies," *FDA Consumer*, May 1990.

9. D. Steinman and S. Epstein, *The Safe Shopper's Bible* (New York: Macmillan, 1995).

10. Steinman and Epstein.

11. J. Linsteadt, "Cosmetics Without Synthetics," Naturalland. Available at www.naturalland.com.

12. Winter.

13. Winter.

14. K. Douthwaite, "Preservatives: Friend or Foe?" *Global Cosmetic Industry*, March 2000.

15. E. Sainio et al., "Metals and Arsenic in Eye Shadows," *Contact Dermatitis* 42 (2000): 5–10.

16. R. Kaltreider et al., "Arsenic Alters the Function of the Glucocorticoid Receptor as a Transcription Factor," *Environmental Health Perspectives* 109 (2001): 245–51.

17. C. Le Cos et al., "Polyvinylpyrrolidone (PVP)/Eicosene Copolymer: An Emerging Cosmetic Allergen," *Contact Dermatitis* 43 (2000): 61–2.

18. "Polyvinylpyrrolidone," MSDS No. P5290, Mallinckrodt Baker, Inc., Phillipsburg, NJ, 8 May 2000.

19. Winter.

20. A. Scheman, "Contact Allergy to Quaternium-22 and Shellac in Mascara," *Contact Dermatitis* 38 (1998): 342–3.

21. Winter.

22. T. Schettler et al., *Generations at Risk* (Cambridge: MIT Press, 1999).

23. Winter.

24. Winter.

25. Y. Nakagawa et al., "Metabolism and Toxicity of Benzophenone in Isolated Rat Hepatocytes and Estrogenic Activity of Its Metabolites in MCF-7 Cells," *Toxicology* 156 (2000): 27–36.

26. "Napthalene," Toxic Chemicals in Your Environment (Technical information sheet), Total Environment Center, Sydney, Australia, 17 Mar 1998.

27. "Tattoos and Permanent Makeup," U.S. Food and Drug Administration Center for Food Safety and Applied Nutrition, Office of Cosmetics and Colors, 29 November 2000.

28. F. Wilson, "Eyelid Tattoo Removal May Require Reconstruction," *Ophthalmology Times*, 1 October 2000.

29. A. Lederberg, "Marked for Life: The Science of Tattoos May Make You Think Before You Ink," *Science World*, 9 March 1998.

30. "FDA Warns Against Use of 'Permanent' Eyelash/Eyebrow Dyes and Tints," U.S. Food and Drug Administration Center for Food Safety and Applied Nutrition, Office of Cosmetics and Colors, 14 July 1992.

31. K. Nash, "Lasers Capable of Removing Makeup Tattoos," *Dermatology Times*, December 1999.

Chapter 10

1. N. Bhatia et al., "Inhibition of Human Carcinoma Cell Growth and DNA Synthesis by Silibinin, an Active Constituent of Milk Thistle: Comparison with Silymarin," *Cancer Letters* 147 (1999): 77–84.

2. R. Gebhardt, "Antioxidant and Protective Properties of Extracts from Leaves of the Artichoke (*Cynara scolymus L.*) Against Hydroperoxide-Induced Oxidative Stress in Cultured Rat Hepatocytes," *Toxicology and Applied Pharmacology* 144 (1997): 279–86.

3. "The New Four Food Groups," Physicians Committee for Responsible Medicine. Available at www.pcrm.org.

4. J. Robbins, *May All Be Fed: Diet for a New World* (New York: William Morrow, 1992).

5. N. Scrimshaw, "An Anaylsis of Past and Present Recommended Dietary Allowances for Protein in Health and Disease," *New England Journal of Medicine*, 22 January 1976. M. Hegsted, "Minimum Protein Requirements of Adults," *American Journal of Clinical Nutrition* 32 (1968): 3520.

6. E. Haas, M.D., founder and director, The Preventive Medical Center of Marin. Telephone interviews with author, January–April 1998.
7. E. Pianin, "Dioxin Report by EPA On Hold," *Washington Post*, 12 April 2001, A01.
8. Campaign to Label Genetically Engineered Foods. Available at www.thecampaign.org.
9. "Organic Food 'Proven' Healthier," BBC News, 3 January 2000. Available at http://newsvote.bbc.co.uk/hi/english/sci tech/newsid'588000/588589.stm.
10. Haas.
11. "Fast Facts on Osteoporosis," National Institutes of Health Osteoporosis and Related Bone Diseases National Resource Center, October 2000. Available at www.osteo.org/osteofastfact.
12. R. Swezey, "Exercise for Osteoporosis: Is Walking Enough? The Case for Site Specificity and Resistive Exercise," *Spine* 21 (1996): 2809–13.

Chapter 11

1. "Stress: America's #1 Health Problem," American Institute of Stress, Yonkers, N.Y. Available at www.stress.org.
2. S. Allen Jr., M.D., clinical assistant professor, State University of New York, Upstate Medical University College of Medicine. Telephone interview with author, 3 March 1996.
3. C. Hassed, "How Humor Keeps You Well," *Australian Family Physician* 30 (2001): 25–8.
4. Dr. J. Goodman, director, The Humor Project, Inc., Saratoga Springs, New York (www.HumorProject.com). Telephone interview with author, 8 March 1996.
5. J. Cameron, *The Artist's Way* (New York: J. P. Tarcher, 1992).
6. R. Steiner, "Some Notes on the 'Heroic Self' and the Meaning and Importance of Its Reparation for the Creative Process and the Creative Personality," *International Journal of Psychoanalysis* 80 (1999): 685–718. R. Helson and J. Pals, "Creative Potential, Creative Achievement, and Personal Growth," *Journal of Personality* 68 (2000): 1–27.
7. B. Dunn et al., "Concentration and Mindfulness Meditations: Unique Forms of Conciousness," *Applied Psychophysiology and Biofeedback* 24 (1999): 147–65.

Index

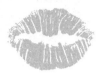